"The Longevity Benefits of Walking"

Walking: The Queen of All Sports

By
Michael Luxiey

CONTENTS

Why Walking is the Queen of all sports? 8

Chapter 1: Physical Health Benefits of Walking.................11

    a. Improved Circulation... 11

    b. Lighten Your Mood 11

    c. Shore Up the Bones...12

    d. It Can Help Lower Your Blood Sugar 12

    e. Extend Your Life! 12

    f. Tone Your Legs 13

    g. Ease Your Eye Strain..13

    h. It Helps Your Aching Body Feel Better....................13

    i. Manage a Wide Range of Diseases 14

    j. A Great Active Recovery 15

    k. Strengthens Muscles...15

Chapter 2: Benefits to Emotional and Mental Health 16

    a) Boosts confidence. 17

    b) Keeps you calm and stress-free. 17

    c) Protects you from various health problems.............17

    d) Improves your memory and concentration.............17

    e) Reconnect with Your Mind and Body.....................18

Chapter 3: The Great Outdoors 19

    a) The Process During the Process 19

    b) Try It Out for Yourself 20

Chapter 4: Neurological Benefits 21

    a) How Walking Improves Self-Esteem......................21

    b) Connecting with Nature 22

    c) Bonding Time with Your Pup 22

d) Using Walking to Connect to the Community 22

e) It's Low-key and Easy to Squeeze In 23

Chapter 5: Identify Things to Make It Better 24

a) Walking for 30 minutes a day 24

b) Make walking part of your routine..25

c) Wear a pedometer while walking. 26

d) A comfortable intensity for walking...26

e) Warming up and cooling down after walking 27

Chapter 6: Making Walking a Pleasure 28

a) Dog Walking...28

b) Walking with Others 29

c) Walking in the Swimming Pool 29

d) Great for All Ability Levels 30

e) Improves Cardio..30

Chapter 7: How Can a Person Get the Most Out of Pool Walking?..32

a) Build Duration Over Time..32

b) Tailor Your Workout 32

c) Use Pool Weights..33

d) Try in Lake or Ocean 33

Chapter 8: Footwear for Walking....................................35

a) How to Select the Right Shoes for Walking 35

b) Shoes for Racewalking 36

c) Shoes for Marathon Walking..37

d) Shoes for Hiking...37

e) What Makes Walking Shoes Different?.......................................38

f) Motion Control Shoes for Overpronators 38

g) What to Wear on a Walk?..39

Chapter 9: Nutrition and Hydration for Walking 42

What to Drink When You Walk 42

A. The importance of proper hydration during walking, including how much water to drink and when to drink it: 44

B. The role of electrolytes in hydration and how to replenish them during long walks: 46

C. The benefits of consuming carbohydrates before a long walk to fuel the body and improve performance. 50

D. The role of protein in recovery after a long walk and how much protein is needed to support muscle repair. 52

E. The importance of consuming a balanced diet that includes fruits, vegetables, whole grains, lean proteins, and healthy fats to support an active lifestyle. 53

F. The benefits of consuming antioxidant-rich foods to reduce inflammation and support recovery after exercise. 55

G. The role of vitamins and minerals in supporting overall health and physical activity, including vitamin D, calcium, and iron. 57

What differentiates the benefits of vitamin D2 from those of vitamin D3? 59

H. Tips for eating on-the-go during long walks, including healthy snack options and portable meals. 61

I. The benefits of meal planning and preparation to ensure that healthy food is readily available for an active lifestyle. 64

J. The importance of consulting a registered dietitian or nutritionist for personalized nutrition and hydration recommendations. 66

Chapter 10: Walking Groups and Communities 70

1- Walking and Community 70

a. Walking groups and clubs 70

b. The benefits of joining these groups 71

c. Tips for finding and joining a walking group. 73

2- Virtual walking communities 74

a. The benefits of joining a virtual walking community 75

b. Virtual walking communities...76

3- Walking events and challenges 81

    a. Walking Events and Challenges....................................82

    b. Training schedules for the events and challenges 87

    c. Tips for participating in these events.................................90

    d. Tips for participating in the Camino del Norte. 90

    e. Nutrition advice 91

    f. Tips for Staying Motivated 92

4- Walking tours and hikes 94

5- Walking for a cause 96

    a. how walking can be used as a tool for advocacy: 96

    b. 10 tips for organizing a fundraising walk: 97

    c. 10 tips for creating a walking challenge for a cause you care about: 98

6- Walking and mental health:..99

Chapter 11: Advanced Walking Techniques 102

    1. Power Walking.. 102

    2. Nordic Walking...106

    3.Interval Walking..109

    4. Figure-Eight Walking or Figure-Eight Walking.................113

Chapter 12: Step by Step: Finding Inspiration and Motivation to Walk 119

    1. Finding the Motivation to Start Walking When You Don't Feel Like It 119

    2. Setting Realistic Goals for Your Walking Routine 122

    3. Tips on how to measure progress and track the benefits of walking include: 124

    4. Making Walking a Social Activity: How to Connect with Others While Exercising.. 128

    5. Incorporating Mindfulness into Your Walking Practice 133

6. Overcoming Obstacles to Consistent Walking: Time, Weather, and Other Challenges..135

7. Incorporating Strength and Stretching Exercises into Your Walking Routine 138

8. Keeping Your Walking Practice Interesting: Exploring New Routes and Techniques... 141

9. Celebrating Your Success: How to Stay Motivated and Reward Yourself Along the Way 143

Chapter 13: Walking Tall: Posture, Safety, and Tips for Every Age and Ability 147

1. What is the Best Time of Day to Walk or Exercise? 147

2. Walking for Weight Loss: 150

3. What If You Can't Walk for 30 Minutes?................................154

4. What About Your Posture? 158

Chapter 14: "Walking Wonders: Real-Life Success Stories in Health Transformation" 164

1. John's Journey to Overcoming Obesity: A Tale of Resilience and Transformation...164

2. Oprah's Story: Managing High Blood Pressure......................166

3. Liam's Story: Overcoming Diabetes 167

4. Walking for Mental Health: Inspiring Stories..........................169

5. In the realm of perpetual unease, Sarah had long been shackled by the chains of anxiety. 172

6. In the relentless whirlwind of workaday chaos, Tom had long been ensnared by the clutches of unyielding stress....................... 175

7. Lila's Story: Walking for Fun and Fitness.............................178

8. Michael's Story: A Quest for Joyful Wellness and Vibrant Living 179

9. Leonardo's Story: Walking for Social Connection 183

10. In the vibrant heart of bustling New York City..................185

11. In the heart of London, we meet Emily 188

12. Italy: "A Walk to Discover Hidden Treasures." 191

13. France: "A Journey of Self-Discovery Through Walking" 193

14. Title: "Tales of Laughter and Leashes: The Adventures of Berlin's Dynamic Dog-Walking Duo" 195

15. Anna had been feeling unmotivated and aimless for months. 199

16. Once upon a time, in the heart of Amsterdam 202

17. In the bustling heart of New York City 205

18. Title: Walking Towards Success in Norway's Challenging Terrain 208

19. Hiking Through the Shadows 211

20. The Camino de Santiago 215

CHAPTER 15: "Globetrotter's Paradise: Unveiling Earth's Most Alluring Walking Trails" **222**

CHAPTER 16: Appendix **234**

1. Famous walkers Throughout History 234

2. Sample Walking Plans...238

3. Glossary of Walking Terms 241

AUTHOR BIO **254**

"The Longevity Benefits of Walking"

Walking: The Secret to a Longer, Healthier Life

Why Walking is the Queen of all sports?

Walking is often referred to as the "queen of all sports" because of its numerous benefits, accessibility, and low impact on the body. While this is an informal title, it highlights the importance and significance of walking as a form of exercise. Here are some reasons why walking might be considered the queen of all sports:

1. Universality: Walking is a natural movement that almost everyone can do, regardless of age, fitness level, or socioeconomic status, making it highly inclusive and accessible.

2. Low impact: Walking is gentle on the joints, making it an ideal exercise for people with joint issues, arthritis, those who are overweight, older individuals, and those recovering from injuries.

3. Health benefits: Walking offers numerous health benefits, including improving cardiovascular health, aiding in weight management, reducing the risk of chronic

diseases such as diabetes and hypertension, and supporting bone health.

4. Mental well-being: Walking has been shown to have a positive impact on mental health by reducing stress, anxiety, and symptoms of depression, and can help improve mood.

5. Enhances creativity and productivity: Walking, especially outdoors, has been linked to increased creativity and clearer thinking, which can lead to new ideas and better problem-solving abilities.

6. Cost-effective: Walking requires minimal equipment – a comfortable pair of shoes is all that is needed – making it an affordable and easily accessible form of exercise for most people.

7. Flexibility: Walking can be done anywhere, anytime, and at any pace, making it easy to incorporate into daily routines or adapt to individual preferences and schedules.

8. Social aspect: Walking can be a social activity, as it's easy to engage in conversation while walking. Many people enjoy walking with friends, family, or in organized walking groups, fostering a sense of community and social connection.

9. Environmental impact: Walking is an eco-friendly form of transportation, as it produces no emissions and requires no fuel. This aspect of

walking aligns with the growing awareness of environmental conservation and sustainability.

10. Longevity: Regular walking has been associated with increased longevity, as it can help to maintain overall health, prevent chronic diseases, and promote a healthy lifestyle.

In summary, walking is considered the "queen of all sports" because of its numerous benefits, accessibility, and adaptability. It's a natural, low-impact, and flexible form of exercise that can be enjoyed by people of all ages and fitness levels, making it an essential component of a healthy lifestyle.

Hippocrates (c. 460 – c. 370 BC): "Walking is the best medicine."

Chapter 1:
Physical Health Benefits of Walking

Here are some of the significant health benefits that you can achieve from walking:

a. Improved Circulation

You will be surprised to know that walking wards off heart disease, raises the heart rate, and strengthens the heart. Postmenopausal women who walk one to two miles a day lower their blood pressure by 11 points in 24 weeks. Research at the Harvard School of Public Health in Boston indicates that women who walk 30 minutes a day can significantly reduce the overall risk of stroke by 20% and 40% when they increase the pace.

b. Lighten Your Mood

Walking also releases natural pain-killing endorphins in the body. It is considered one of the emotional benefits of exercise. A study at California State University showed that the more steps people took during the day, the better their moods.

To experience this benefit, aim for 30 minutes of brisk walking as well as another moderate-intensity exercise three days a week. You also have the option to break it up into three 10-minute walks, depending on your preference.

c. Shore Up the Bones

According to Michael A. Schwartz, walking is responsible for halting bone mass loss for people who have osteoporosis. In fact, another study of postmenopausal women found that half an hour of walking daily significantly reduced the overall risk of hip fractures by 40%.

d. It Can Help Lower Your Blood Sugar

Taking a walk after eating significantly aids in lowering blood sugar. A study suggests that taking a 15-minute walk three times a day, especially after meals, significantly improves blood sugar levels compared to taking a 45-minute walk during the day. However, further research is required to confirm these findings. For optimal results, consider making a post-meal walk a part of your routine, as it also helps incorporate exercise throughout the day.

e. Extend Your Life!

Recent research indicates that people who exercise daily in their fifties and sixties are 35% less likely to die over the next eight years compared to their non-walking counterparts. However, this number increases to 45% for those with underlying health conditions.

Moreover, walking at a faster pace can also extend life. Brisk walking reduces the risk of death by 24 percent. Scientific studies have examined the association of walking at a quicker pace with factors such as overall causes of death, death from cancer, and cardiovascular disease.

f. Tone Your Legs

Walking also strengthens the muscles in the legs. To build more strength, walk on a treadmill with an incline or find routes with stairs. Additionally, consider integrating cross-training activities such as cycling or jogging. You can also perform resistance exercises such as squats, lunges, and leg curls to further tone and strengthen leg muscles.

g. Ease Your Eye Strain

Staring at a screen all day narrows the range of focus to a few feet in front, causing fatigue in the eye muscles. This contributes to digital eye strain and focus issues. While it typically doesn't harm vision in the long run, it may cause symptoms like headaches, sore eyes, or blurred vision.

Walking outdoors requires the use of long-range vision and constant scaling of obstacles. The more you observe your surroundings, the better the brain and eyes work together for processing.

h. It Helps Your Aching Body Feel Better

It's essential to note that walking gives the body a break from intense training, which can prevent overuse injuries. Additionally, walking is an effective way to manage various aches. A recent study published in the journal Evidence-Based Practice found that walking was more effective than physical therapy in treating low back pain among 246 adults.

To reap these benefits, maintaining proper form is crucial. Many strides have adapted to years of injuries, leading many people to lean forward. To offset some of this strain, try using therapy balls to roll the body beforehand, and incorporate a warm-up routine including bodyweight squats, forward folds, and lunges.

i. Manage a Wide Range of Diseases

Think of any health benefit associated with exercise, and chances are there is research showing walking can help achieve it. A scientific study published in Creative Nursing reports that just ten weeks of walking for 20 minutes daily improved women's blood pressure and cholesterol.

Moreover, for individuals with illnesses or chronic conditions, walking is more accessible compared to other forms of exercise and can still provide significant benefits like improved function, reduced fatigue during breast cancer treatment, better blood sugar control, and increased quality of life.

j. A Great Active Recovery

Every high-intensity interval comes with a recovery period. Walking keeps the muscles warm and the heart pumping. You can also incorporate some steps between strength movements to add a low-impact cardio boost.

Regular walking serves as an active recovery session on days when high-intensity workouts are not feasible. This not only gives the body a break but may also speed up recovery by enhancing blood flow to sore and tired muscles.

k. Strengthens Muscles

Walking tones both leg and abdominal muscles and pumping your arms as you walk can engage arm muscles as well. It increases your range of motion, shifting pressure and weight from joints to muscles. Recent scientific studies have found that women aged 50 to 75 who took a one-hour walk were more likely to relieve insomnia compared to women who didn't walk.

Gary Snyder (1930): "Walking is a great adventure, the first meditation, a practice of heartiness and soul primary to humankind. Walking is the exact balance between spirit and humility."

Chapter 2:
Benefits to Emotional and Mental Health

Walking offers benefits beyond just physical health; it also enhances mental and emotional well-being. Even a 15-minute walk can provide substantial benefits in these areas. Are you struggling to make walking a priority in your self-care? If so, let's find out how walking can benefit you mentally and emotionally.

It is fascinating to know that walking helps boost the mind, mood, and emotional well-being. The reason is that regular walking is responsible for increasing blood circulation and blood flow to both the body and brain. Walking shows a positive influence on the hypothalamic-pituitary-adrenal (HPA) axis, which is called your central nervous response system. It is best because the HPA axis is responsible for the stress response. However, when you exercise by walking, you directly calm the nerves that make you feel less stressed.

Furthermore, one of the best ways to reap the benefits of walking is by inviting friends to join you. Walking with companions for one or two days a week can have significant advantages. Physical exercise with positive social interactions improves negative moods. In this way, you can significantly get rid of depression, stress, and anxiety. Walking improves self-esteem.

a) Boosts confidence.

By improving stamina and endurance levels, you will have tremendous confidence in walking faster for better workouts.

b) Keeps you calm and stress-free.

If you find yourself working overtime or for extended hours, be sure to take short breaks to move around every half-hour. This will help alleviate tiredness and keep you energized and stress-free in challenging situations.

c) Protects you from various health problems.

An inactive or sedentary lifestyle leads to multiple health risks. By walking regularly, you not only improve your mood, but you can also stay safe from numerous diseases and illnesses that are directly related to a lack of mobility and exercise, such as cardiac ailments, stroke, low blood pressure levels, diabetes, and most importantly, obesity.

d) Improves your memory and concentration.

Doctors have reported that even a brief 10-minute brisk walk can quickly improve brain function. Researchers have also observed that people had improved concentration and memory in specific areas of their minds that functioned better in various memory tests after the workout.

e) Reconnect with Your Mind and Body

If walking continuously for sixty minutes is challenging, consider taking shorter, more frequent walks instead. Taking small breaks to walk during work can make you feel more energized. It is essential to note that walking supports the production of endorphins responsible for reducing anxiety levels. Walking also helps avoid unnecessary stressors and aids in reconnecting with your mind and body.

Charles Dickens (1812-1870): "The sum of the whole is this: walk and be happy; walk and be healthy."

Chapter 3:
The Great Outdoors

When you walk outside, you experience the added benefits of being in nature. Walking outdoors means you are going to spend an extraordinary amount of time outside. In this era of digital technology, the lack of fresh air and limited exposure to natural light are problematic aspects of contemporary lifestyles. Spending more time in the fresh air increases energy and improves mood. Additionally, natural light plays an essential role in the biological clocks responsible for regulating the level of hormones and sleep cycles. Night light exposure reduces the depressive symptoms caused by seasonal affective disorder (SAD).

According to scientific studies, walking has been shown to improve overall mood. Furthermore, nature also plays a vital role in connecting people to the more fantastic world. Furthermore, being in nature allows you to immerse yourself in the outside world, improving mood and fostering a sense of connection.

a) The Process During the Process
When you walk, you increase overall productivity, creativity, as well as access to emotions. It is fascinating to know that regular walking has been shown to boost the free flow of ideas, as well as your sense of creativity and inspiration. Research has shown an increase in

productivity following a brief walk. Finally, walking plays an essential role in connecting you with your body. As a result, you become more aware of your emotions, especially when feeling overwhelmed.

b) Try It Out for Yourself

Undoubtedly, scientific research is clear that there are many mental health benefits to walking. However, one of the best ways to gauge the positive benefits of walking is for you to try it yourself. Find some time that is just for yourself; it can be as little as 15 minutes. You can go somewhere you find relaxing. Before you start walking, rate your mood on a scale of 1 (terrible) to 10 (outstanding). When you finish the walk, rate your mood again; the slight uptick in mood is significant. Another way to gauge the impact of walking is to focus on a mental problem while walking. You can use this framework for thinking about a feeling that can be confusing to you. At the end of the walk, reassess the problem. Chances are you will have an alternative view of it. Take some time out of your day to go for a walk and notice how beneficial daily walks can be for you.

Mahatma Gandhi (1869-1948): "I believe that there is a subtle magnetism in Nature, which, if we unconsciously yield to it, will direct us a right."

Chapter 4:
Neurological Benefits

When you walk, there are some neurochemical changes that happen which significantly and positively impact your mood. Any type of active movement, such as walking, increases endorphins as well as norepinephrine. This is important to consider because endorphins are regarded as one of the significant contributors to feelings of happiness and euphoria. It is the reason why people report a boost in mood after engaging in physical activity.

On the flip side, norepinephrine is the neurochemical that plays an essential role in the brain's response to stress. Engaging in regular walking can significantly decrease current stress levels and help the brain effectively handle future stress responses. Furthermore, a neurological bonus of walking is that it also prevents cognitive decline by increasing the chemicals that support the hippocampus. The hippocampus is the primary essential part of the brain that plays a role in learning and memory.

a) How Walking Improves Self-Esteem

Walking can improve self-esteem. When you are around negative people or people who want to bring you down, it can lower your self-esteem. When you notice that your self-esteem is dropping, it is the best time to take action. If you choose to walk regularly, it will make you feel good inside. The reason is that the metabolic rate starts producing energy, promoting good health. However, any exercise builds your self-esteem and boosts confidence.

b) Connecting with Nature

People have an inherent relationship with the natural world, and walking in a park or near a body of water makes you feel more centered. Compared to a busy road, forest walking plays a significant role in providing psychological benefits.

c) Bonding Time with Your Pup

The average dog owner walks an extra 22 minutes daily. A British study of 43 pairs of dog owners, as well as non-dog owners, found that this seems enough to reap health benefits for you and your pup. Walking helps your pet's joints, weight, digestion, and behavior. It is also a fun way to spend quality time with your dog, whether you are one of those who adopted a pandemic puppy or not.

d) Using Walking to Connect to the Community

Many people are not traveling these days. For them, walking offers the best chance to act like a tourist in their neighborhood. In this situation, you have the best chance to visit the outdoor attractions that you never get a chance to check out. You can find a new path and name it a secret garden. While walking, you have the best opportunity to forge deeper bonds with your friends or neighbors. Walking has become more crucial than ever in light of the side effects of COVID-19. You have the best opportunity to stride door-to-door to check in from a distance with neighbors who are outdoors, carry food, and other supplies to the needy people.

e) It's Low-key and Easy to Squeeze In

Unlike other exercises, you will not get sweaty during the walk, which means there is no need to schedule a shower during the workday. However, if you are working from home, a regular walk offers a welcome escape. It is fascinating to know that there is no need to change clothes: swap the slippers and work shoes for walking shoes. You can use brisk walking to run errands and warm up before engaging in another physical activity.

John Muir (1838-1914): "Keep close to Nature's heart... and break clear away, once in a while, and climb a mountain or spend a week in the woods. Wash your spirit clean."

Chapter 5:
Identify Things to Make It Better

If you are new to strolling around the community and are now checking out what it has to offer, you may realize that it might be a fertile breeding ground to identify things that could benefit from some change. As you stride, you can look out for places that need attention, such as a route that needs bright lighting, a busy street that requires a crosswalk, or a path. After that, send requests for improvements straight to the city council representative and the park district chairperson. Along with this, you can check online groups for neighborhoods, such as via Facebook or Nextdoor, to see if anyone has already flagged the issue.

Whether you are taking to the streets to improve your community, boost fitness, or calm your thoughts, adding a daily walk is a feel-good change to the routine. Just consider it an act of fitness self-care for both the mind and the body.

a) Walking for 30 minutes a day

To get the health benefits, walk for 30 minutes as briskly as you can. A brisk walk means you can talk but not sing during the walk, and you may be puffing slightly. Moderate activities like walking pose little health risk. However, if you have any medical conditions, check with your doctor before starting any exercise program.

If walking for 30 minutes seems complicated, consider breaking it into smaller, more manageable bouts three times a day. You can also gradually build up for longer sessions. If the goal is to lose weight, you need to do physical activity for more than 30 minutes daily. Yes, you still have a chance to achieve this by starting with more minor bouts of exercise to improve your fitness level.

b) Make walking part of your routine.
It would be best to make walking a part of your routine. Keep in mind that you are using the same amount of energy, no matter what time of day you are walking. You will find that asking someone to walk with you will help make it a regular activity. Physical activity in any form can be built into a lifestyle plan, which is one of the best ways to assist with weight loss and weight maintenance. Some suggestions for building walking into your daily life include:

Take the stairs instead of the lift.
Get off public transport one stop early and walk to work and home.
Walk to the local shops.
Walk with your dog!

c) Wear a pedometer while walking.

A pedometer is used to measure the number of steps you take. It is best to use a pedometer to count your movement throughout the day and compare it to other days. It will motivate you to move more. However, the recommended number of steps per day in order to achieve health benefits is 10,000 steps or more.

d) A comfortable intensity for walking

Many people think there's little difference in the energy expended when walking a kilometer compared to running one because walking takes longer. You can plan to cover a set distance daily and monitor how long it takes to walk this distance. As your fitness level gradually improves, you will walk a longer distance and use more energy. Brisk walking burns more calories than walking slowly, but it doesn't mean you have to push yourself until you are breathless. Pace yourself so that you can talk. The simple rule of thumb means you have to walk safely within the target heart rate that brings about health gains.

Moreover, human bodies tend to get used to physical activity. You can continue walking to increase the intensity as you are capable of improving your fitness levels. However, you can increase the power of your walks by:

Walking up hills

Increasing the walking speed gradually by adding some quick walking

Increasing the distance

Walking with hand weights

Walking for longer

e) Warming up and cooling down after walking

An excellent way to warm up is to walk slowly. It is suggested to start a walk at a leisurely pace to give the muscles the best time to warm up and then pick up the speed. Then, gently stretch your leg muscles as well as your calves and front and back thighs. Stretching must be held for about 20 seconds. If you feel pain, ease off the stretch. Overstretching your muscle tissue can cause microscopic tears.

You should dress lightly while doing physical activity. Dressing warmly can increase sweating. It also raises body temperature, making you uncomfortable during a walk. It's good to know that a gradual cool-down also prevents injury and muscle stiffness.

Henry David Thoreau (1817-1862): "An early-morning walk is a blessing for the whole day."

Chapter 6:
Making Walking a Pleasure

Some recommendations for making regular walking a pleasurable form of physical activity are:

Varying where you walk
Walking the dog
Walking with friends
Joining a walking club

a) Dog Walking

A dog that needs exercise can also motivate you to walk every day. You may enjoy the companionship, too. However, if you don't have a dog, consider offering to walk a neighbor's dog.

However, some suggestions for the safety of the dog and other pedestrians are:

Be considerate of other pedestrians. Always keep the dog on its leash.

If you are planning to walk in a park, check if dogs are allowed. Several national and state parks do not permit dogs.

Other parks may permit dog walking on a leash.

Take equipment like plastic bags and gloves to clean up after your dog.

b) Walking with Others

Walking with other people can turn your exercise into an enjoyable social occasion. Suggestions are:

Schedule a regular family walk. It is considered the best way to pass on healthy habits to children and grandchildren while spending time together.

If you are walking with children, ensure that the route and length of walking time are appropriate for their age.

Babies or toddlers enjoy long walks in the pram. You can take the opportunity to point out items of interest to young ones.

Look for self-guided nature walks in many parks. Some younger children enjoy looking for the next numbered post, while older children can learn about the plants and animals in the garden.

Ask your neighbors and friends if they would like to join you on your walks.

c) Walking in the Swimming Pool

Many people think of swimming pool running as the primary way to exercise in a pool. However, pool walking can be a great option. As a go-to workout for physical therapists and trainers, pool walking is as straightforward or as complicated as needed. Let's have a look at how pool walking is considered a valuable part of the exercise routine.

d) Great for All Ability Levels

The diversity in workouts makes it a beneficial option for people of all fitness levels. However, it can be as easy as walking in the pool's shallow end or as complex as high-intensity interval training. It is important to note that pool walking is done in shallow water with feet touching the bottom of the pool. Many weights and resistance-training exercises are incorporated into pool-walking workouts.

Along with this, water workouts offer different advantages compared to land workouts. As water is buoyant, people with joint issues are more comfortable working out in the water. It is also a good option for people with high training volumes in running and weightlifting as water provides resistance to help tone muscles naturally.

e) Improves Cardio

It is important to know that pool-walking workouts can be as long or short as you like. However, 20–45 minutes is considered a reasonable length of time to get the heart rate up and in the zone that permits you to work on cardiovascular health.

Pool workouts are fantastic ways to work on stability and balance that are beneficial for everyone, especially for those recovering from an injury. The water helps with the range of motion, and you can push the limits of balance in the water.

Helen Keller (1880-1968): "Walking has always been a part of my life, and it still is today. Just as the water feeds the body and spirit, the sight of trees and flowers nourishes the eyes."

Chapter 7:
How Can a Person Get the Most Out of Pool Walking?

a) Build Duration Over Time

Pool walking may feel easy at the moment, and it's common to overdo it. It would be best to start easily and gradually build up the duration, intensity, or frequency. Ensure to record the workouts in a journal with how you felt afterward. It will help you a lot in determining whether the pool workouts are working for you and how to adjust to see the most success.

b) Tailor Your Workout

Although pool walking is commonly used to rehabilitate from injuries, it doesn't mean that it cannot be used as a tool for advanced athletes. You can make pool walking as difficult or easy as required by using the guidelines below:

To make it harder:

Increase the duration.
Increase the speed.
Go deeper into the pool.
Walk against a current.
Wear special webbed gloves that make it harder for you to pump your arms through the water.
Perform Tabata-style high-intensity sessions.

To make it easier:

Slow the pace.
Take more frequent rest breaks.
Do a shorter workout.
Avoid water with a current.
Stay in the shallow area.
Work on Your Balance

People do a lot of work in the pool, such as standing on one foot and moving from side to side and leaning forward or backward as you walk, which helps improve stability on land. It is suitable for anyone with an injury who is unable to do balance work on the ground and wants to improve balance in general or for a specific sport such as skiing or surfing.

c) Use Pool Weights

Adding weights to the pool workout has significant benefits, whether you walk with them in your hands or do resistance-training exercises. The wide range of motion in the pool is more prominent because the water supports you, meaning that you will sit more profoundly in a squat and reach further overhead in the water.

d) Try in Lake or Ocean

The benefits of exercising outdoors are well-documented. However, if you can, take the water-walking workout to a natural body of water. It seems like a challenging activity because the water is about thigh-deep and drags on your legs.

John Muir (1838-1914): "In every walk with nature, one receives far more than he seeks."

Chapter 8:
Footwear for Walking

It is fascinating to know that walking is a low-cost as well as an effective form of exercise. However, the wrong type of shoe and walking action can cause foot or shin pain, blisters, or injuries to soft tissue. Before walking, ensure that your shoes are comfortable, with the right heel and arch supports. Take it light with easy steps. While walking, make sure that your heels touch down before your toes. It would be best to walk on grass rather than concrete to absorb the impact.

a) How to Select the Right Shoes for Walking

Times have changed now, and today there are a variety of shoes for every activity. But why? Do walkers need different shoes for strolling vs. racewalking as well as hiking? Does it matter? Well, in a word, yes.

Bear in mind that all walkers were not created equal. Just as Cenedella's slipper fit only her foot, your shoes fit only one fitness activity. Various ways of walking require multiple types of shoe designs as well as materials. Along with this, the overall lightness and flexibility of a racewalking shoe can spell disaster on a challenging hike.

For casual fitness walking, anything goes, as opposed to racewalkers who are planning to cover three to five miles at a time with real racewalking shoes. Walkers impact the ground with less than half the force of runners. It means they don't need excessive cushioning. There is a great need to know that too much fluff in the heel may lead to shin pain or other problems. A good rule of the big toe is that any comfortable running, walking, and racewalking shoe that cannot give you blisters is okay for casual walking.

b) Shoes for Racewalking

Increasing fitness and competitive activity, racewalking is not only fast walking. Keep in mind, Olympic style racewalking uses more muscles and relies on the feet than fitness walking does. For this purpose, the right pair of shoes is essential.

Racewalking shoes also require being flexible to allow the feet to roll from heel to toe. It is fascinating to know that these shoes must have a shallow heel to reduce the leverage that causes the feet to slap the ground after the direct contact of the heel. Authentic racewalking shoes or running racing flats are your best bets.

c) Shoes for Marathon Walking

Walking marathons, as well as even three-day ultra-marathons, are another type of athletic challenge. Marathon walking is getting popular day by day. How you walk one of these events dictates what you should wear.

A lot of marathon walkers use simple fitness walking techniques. For this purpose, walking shoes or lightweight running shoes are best. However, a growing number of marathons also include competitive racewalking. If you are planning on racewalking a marathon, you will need a good racewalking shoe.

Picking the perfect pair of shoes is essential, but the fit of these shoes is one of the most critical factors when you are on your feet for several hours. Shoes that are tight or loose can cause painful blisters.

d) Shoes for Hiking

Hiking shoes are all about disaster avoidance. For most hikes, anything with a treaded and high-grip outsole will do. People also wear a pair of sandals for easy hikes, but for more rugged terrain, there is a need to invest in something substantial to prevent ankle sprains.

If you want to buy fitness walking shoes or hiking boots, they are available in most athletic shoe stores as well as online. However, flats and racewalking might be challenging to find.

e) What Makes Walking Shoes Different?

No matter how great a shoe looks, it won't do you any good if it doesn't fit properly. To ensure a good fit, it's best to find the best athletic shoe store in your area. Personal trainers are an excellent resource for this. Always make sure to keep an eye out for stores that provide foot analysis, as it is an indication that they'll be able to find a shoe that is anatomically suited to your foot. Walking shoes are different from running shoes in every aspect of how a person moves. Walkers strike first with the heel and roll through the step.

f) Motion Control Shoes for Overpronators

If you overpronate, you need to get a pair of motion control shoes to compensate. This is especially true if you are heavy or have other mobility issues, such as a weak knee or hip. Keep in mind that motion control shoes are more severe, as they offer firmer support. These shoes help balance the gait while walking.

When searching for the right walking shoe, there is no need to get hung up on labels. If you have found a flexible, flat shoe, it may be well-suited for walking, even if it's labeled as a running shoe. Numerous walking shoes have bells and whistles.

If you want to make the best choice, place function before fashion. You want to look great, but it's crucial to find something that makes walking a joy. You can easily find a great pair of shoes between $60 and $120.

g) What to Wear on a Walk?

It significantly depends on the type of walk you are going on, as well as the weather conditions. For easy access walks on good paths with good weather, you can get away with regular clothing, as long as it's comfortable. However, a leisurely walk around town in walking gear will probably lead to you getting funny looks.

As you progress to more leisurely or strenuous walks, you need to wear appropriate clothing as the weather conditions worsen. In mountainous areas, the weather is changeable, and you must bring clothing with you that is suitable for a range of weather conditions. If it seems like a lovely sunny day while leaving the house, it might be raining and windy at the top of the mountain.

Here are some tips on what to bring:

1. Bring a sturdy and supportive pair of walking boots. For walkers, these should be worn appropriately.

2. It would be best if you brought an excellent windproof coat. If the weather is terrible, you will almost certainly get wet, and there will be a need for a coat that keeps the wind off.

3. Bring a series of comfortable, thin layers that can be worn and removed as needed.

4. You can also bring a good pair of gloves with a hat to keep the extremities warm.

5. You should try to use technical clothing that dries quickly.

6. In areas or countries where hot sunny days are less common, if it looks like the sun might make an appearance, bring a sun hat and wear lighter clothing.

7. Do not wear cotton or denim while walking. The reason is that cotton draws heat from the body when it is wet and causes you to get cold if you have layers on top of the cotton. On the flip side, denim stays wet

for a long time, which may cause your legs to get cold.

8. Waterproof trousers and waterproof socks can be helpful when the weather is terrible.

It is essential to keep in mind that a poor clothing choice is considered one of the best ways to ruin a day's walk, and it might be potentially fatal. Ensure that any clothing you are not wearing is stored somewhere waterproof, and there is no point in bringing spare clothes if they are sodden before you put them on. There is no need to spend money to start. For a walk, you can start with casual dressing by keeping the weather in mind.

Chapter 9:
Nutrition and Hydration for Walking

What to Drink When You Walk

We all know that it's essential to stay hydrated when we work out or have a long walk. However, we may not be so clear on what exactly we should drink when we walk or exercise.

Ordinary water is the classic choice. However, with sports drinks, energy drinks, and various flavored and fortified water drinks lining store shelves everywhere, we have more options than ever before. According to the experts, the choice significantly depends on your workout's length, intensity, and taste.

If you find that you drink more when your beverage is flavored, it's better to choose whatever helps you stay hydrated during your walk or exercise. Water is considered the best form of hydration, and for endurance, some sports drinks can be effective at getting the body to absorb fluid quickly. Unlike sports drinks, energy drinks are not a good source of hydration in endurance activities, where hydration is paramount.

You might be just as happy with dressed-up regular water, with the option to flavor it with lemon, lime, orange, or a strawberry or two. However, green tea is also a healthy choice for you. It may be unconventional, but green tea is considered a healthy way to consume fluids daily. When it comes to sports drinks, they offer the body three essential things it needs before, during, and after the walk:

Hydration: The American College of Sports Medicine suggests that people drink about 17 ounces of fluid two hours before a workout to promote hydration. It also allows the body to excrete excess water, so you may not feel any difficulty during the walk or any other exercise. During exercise, it is recommended that people start drinking early at regular intervals to take in fluids at the rate they are losing.

Fuel: It's important to note that the carbohydrates found in sweetened sports drinks provide the energy to combat fatigue. Tests have shown that a 6% carbohydrate solution is the optimal percentage for speeding up fluid and fuel absorption into the body.

Minerals or Electrolytes: These include sodium, potassium, and chloride. Athletes and intensive walkers lose these minerals through sweat. When the body is losing water, it makes sense to replace electrolytes.

Here are some general guidelines:

Before the walk: Try to start hydrating two hours before the planned activity by aiming for a fluid intake of 5 to 6 milliliters per kilogram of body weight.

During the walk: If you are exercising for an hour and in warm weather, find a fluid replacement beverage that contains sodium, potassium, and carbohydrates for maximum hydration.

After the walk: You can consume sports beverages or drink water as well as eat foods that contain sodium for proper rehydration. For each kilogram of body weight lost during a brisk walk, slowly consume 1.5 liters of fluid.

A. The importance of proper hydration during walking, including how much water to drink and when to drink it:

Proper hydration during walking is essential for maintaining good health and preventing dehydration. When you walk, your body sweats to regulate body temperature and this results in the loss of water and electrolytes. Dehydration can lead to fatigue, dizziness, muscle cramps, and other serious health problems. Therefore, it is important to drink enough water to replace the fluids lost during walking.

How much water to drink during walking depends on several factors such as your body weight, the temperature and humidity of the environment, and the intensity and duration of your walk. As a general guideline, it is recommended to drink about 17-20 ounces (500-600 ml) of water two to three hours before walking to hydrate your body, and then 7-10 ounces (200-300 ml) of water every 10-20 minutes during your walk. If you are walking for longer than an hour, you may need to drink more water to prevent dehydration.

It is also important to listen to your body's signals and drink water when you feel thirsty. Thirst is a sign of mild dehydration, so if you feel thirsty during your walk, it is time to take a break and drink some water.

In addition to water, you can also drink other fluids that contain electrolytes such as sports drinks, coconut water, or fruit juices to help replenish the minerals lost during sweating. However, be mindful of the sugar content in these drinks, as excessive consumption of sugary drinks can lead to weight gain and other health issues.

In conclusion, proper hydration during walking is crucial for maintaining good health and preventing dehydration. It is important to drink enough water before, during, and after your walk, and to listen to your body's signals to prevent dehydration.

B. The role of electrolytes in hydration and how to replenish them during long walks:

Electrolytes are minerals that help regulate fluid balance in your body and are important for proper hydration. They include sodium, potassium, magnesium, calcium, and chloride. During long walks, your body loses electrolytes through sweat, and it is important to replenish them to maintain optimal hydration and prevent cramping, fatigue, and other health problems.

To replenish electrolytes during long walks, you can consume foods and drinks that are high in these minerals. Here are some options:

1. Sports drinks: These drinks are specifically formulated to replace electrolytes lost during exercise. Look for drinks that contain sodium, potassium, and magnesium, and avoid those that are high in sugar. Most sports drinks contain around 110-170 milligrams of sodium per 8-ounce serving, along with smaller amounts of potassium, magnesium, and calcium.

2. Coconut Water: A natural hydrating option, coconut water boasts significant amounts of potassium and magnesium, with lower sugar content compared to numerous sports drinks. A serving of one cup (240 ml) provides

approximately 480 milligrams of potassium, 30 milligrams of sodium, and 57 milligrams of magnesium.

3. Bananas: This fruit is rich in potassium, making it a great option for replenishing electrolytes. One medium-sized banana contains about 400-450 milligrams of potassium.

4. Leafy greens: Vegetables such as spinach, kale, and broccoli are good sources of calcium, magnesium, and potassium. One cup of raw spinach contains about 167 milligrams of calcium, 24 milligrams of magnesium, and 167 milligrams of potassium.

5. Nuts and seeds: Almonds, pumpkin seeds, and sunflower seeds are high in magnesium, while pistachios are a useful source of potassium. One ounce (28 grams) of almonds contains about 75 milligrams of calcium and 80 milligrams of magnesium, while one ounce of pumpkin seeds contains about 150 milligrams of magnesium and 130 milligrams of potassium.

6. Electrolyte tablets: These tablets can be dissolved in water and provide a concentrated dose of electrolytes.

7. Watermelon: This juicy fruit is a good source of potassium and magnesium, and also contains high amounts of water to help with hydration. One cup of diced watermelon contains about 170 milligrams of potassium and seventeen milligrams of calcium.

8. Tomatoes: These red, juicy fruits are high in potassium, making them a fantastic addition to a post-walk meal. One medium-sized tomato contains about 290 milligrams of potassium, 10 milligrams of sodium, and 24 milligrams of magnesium.

9. Yogurt: This dairy product is rich in calcium and potassium and can help replenish electrolytes after a walk. One 8-ounce serving of plain low-fat yogurt contains about 400 milligrams of calcium and 520 milligrams of potassium.

10. Celery: This crunchy vegetable is high in sodium and potassium and can be a refreshing snack during a long walk. One cup of chopped celery contains about 40 milligrams of sodium, 260 milligrams of potassium, and 16 milligrams of calcium.

11. Pickles: These salty snacks are high in sodium, making them a good option for replenishing electrolytes lost through sweat. One medium-sized pickle contains about 220 milligrams of sodium.

12. Herbal tea: Certain types of herbal teas, such as nettle tea and dandelion root tea, can help replenish electrolytes and provide other health benefits as well. The electrolyte content of herbal tea can vary depending on the type of tea. For example, nettle tea is high in calcium, magnesium, and potassium, while dandelion root tea is high in potassium.

It is important to consume these foods and drinks in moderation and to balance them with water to avoid overconsumption of electrolytes, which can be harmful. Additionally, it's important to be mindful of the sugar content in sports drinks and other beverages, as excessive sugar consumption can lead to weight gain and other health problems.

Again, these are just rough estimates, and can vary depending on the type and variety of the food or drink. It is also important to remember that electrolyte needs can vary widely depending on individual factors, such as age, sex, body size, and activity level. Therefore, it is best to consult with a healthcare provider or registered dietitian to determine your specific electrolyte needs and develop a personalized hydration strategy.

In conclusion, electrolytes play a crucial role in hydration, and it is important to replenish them during long walks to maintain optimal health. Consuming foods and drinks that are high in electrolytes, such as sports drinks, coconut water, bananas, leafy greens, nuts, and seeds, can help you maintain proper electrolyte balance during exercise.

C. The benefits of consuming carbohydrates before a long walk to fuel the body and improve performance.

Consuming carbohydrates before a long walk can provide several benefits, including improved fueling for the body and enhanced performance. Here are some of the main benefits of consuming carbohydrates before a long walk:

1. Increased energy: Carbohydrates are the primary source of energy for the body, so consuming them before a long walk can provide a boost of energy to help you power through your walk.

2. Improved endurance: Consuming carbohydrates before a long walk can help delay the onset of fatigue and improve endurance,

allowing you to walk for longer periods of time without feeling tired.

3.   Better glycogen storage: Carbohydrates are stored in the body as glycogen, which is used to fuel physical activity. By consuming carbohydrates before a long walk, you can help ensure that your glycogen stores are fully stocked and ready to provide energy for your walk.

4.   Faster recovery: Consuming carbohydrates before a long walk can also help speed up the recovery process after your walk, as glycogen stores are depleted during physical activity and need to be replenished.

Some good carbohydrate-rich foods to consume before a long walk include whole grain bread, pasta, rice, oatmeal, fruit, and vegetables. Aim to consume your pre-walk meal at least one to three hours before your walk to allow time for digestion and be sure to hydrate well with water and electrolytes. Additionally, it is important to find the right balance of carbohydrates for your individual needs, as too many or too few carbohydrates can have negative effects on performance.

D. The role of protein in recovery after a long walk and how much protein is needed to support muscle repair.

Protein plays a crucial role in recovery after a long walk, as it helps repair and rebuild muscle tissue that may have been damaged during the activity. Here are some of the main ways protein supports muscle recovery after a long walk:

1. Muscle repair: When you engage in physical activity such as walking, your muscles can become damaged and may require repair. Protein provides the building blocks necessary to repair and rebuild muscle tissue, helping to prevent soreness and promote recovery.

2. Improved muscle growth: Consuming protein after a long walk can also help promote muscle growth and improve overall strength, which can be beneficial for future physical activity.

3. Increased satiety: Protein is also more filling than carbohydrates or fats, which can help reduce hunger and prevent overeating after a long walk.

The amount of protein needed to support muscle repair after a long walk can vary depending on a number of factors, including your body weight, age, sex, and activity level. However, a general rule of thumb is to consume around 20-30 grams of protein within 30 minutes to an hour after your walk. Some useful sources of protein for muscle recovery include lean meats, poultry, fish, eggs, dairy products, legumes, nuts, and seeds.

It's also important to note that protein alone is not enough to support muscle recovery after a long walk. Adequate hydration and carbohydrate intake are also important for optimal recovery, as carbohydrates provide the energy needed for physical activity and hydration helps with nutrient delivery and waste removal. Therefore, it's important to maintain a well-balanced diet that includes a variety of nutrient-rich foods to support your body's recovery after physical activity.

E. The importance of consuming a balanced diet that includes fruits, vegetables, whole grains, lean proteins, and healthy fats to support an active lifestyle.

Consuming a balanced diet that includes a variety of nutrient-rich foods is crucial for supporting an active lifestyle and promoting overall health and well-being. Here are some of the key benefits of consuming a balanced diet:

1. Improved energy levels: Consuming a balanced diet that includes a mix of carbohydrates, protein, and healthy fats can provide the energy needed to power through physical activity and maintain energy levels throughout the day.

2. Enhanced nutrient intake: Consuming a variety of fruits, vegetables, whole grains, lean proteins, and healthy fats can help ensure that you are getting all of the essential nutrients needed for optimal health and performance, including vitamins, minerals, and antioxidants.

3. Improved recovery: Consuming a balanced diet that includes protein, carbohydrates, and healthy fats can help support muscle recovery after physical activity, reduce inflammation, and promote optimal immune function.

4. Reduced risk of chronic disease: Consuming a diet that is high in nutrient-rich foods can help reduce the risk of chronic diseases such as heart disease, diabetes, and certain types of cancer.

5. To support an active lifestyle, focus on consuming a variety of nutrient-rich foods such as:

6. Fruits and vegetables: Aim for a variety of colors and types, as each provides unique vitamins, minerals, and antioxidants.

7. Whole grains: Choose whole grains such as brown rice, quinoa, and whole wheat bread for fiber, vitamins, and minerals.

8. Lean proteins: Include sources of lean protein such as chicken, fish, tofu, and legumes to support muscle repair and growth.

9. Healthy fats: Incorporate sources of healthy fats such as avocado, nuts, seeds, and olive oil to support brain function and reduce inflammation.

10. By consuming a balanced diet that includes a variety of nutrient-rich foods, you can support your body's needs for physical activity and promote optimal health and well-being.

F. The benefits of consuming antioxidant-rich foods to reduce inflammation and support recovery after exercise.

Consuming antioxidant-rich foods can provide several benefits for reducing inflammation and supporting recovery after exercise. Here are some of the key benefits:

1. Reduced inflammation: Exercise can cause temporary inflammation in the body as part of the process of muscle repair and growth.

However, chronic inflammation can be harmful to overall health and can interfere with recovery. Antioxidants help reduce inflammation by neutralizing free radicals, which are unstable molecules that can damage cells and contribute to inflammation.

2. Improved recovery: Consuming antioxidant-rich foods can also help support recovery after exercise by reducing muscle damage and soreness. Antioxidants have been shown to help reduce muscle damage caused by exercise and promote muscle repair and recovery.

3. Reduced oxidative stress: Exercise can also increase oxidative stress in the body, which can contribute to inflammation and damage to cells. Antioxidants help reduce oxidative stress by neutralizing free radicals and protecting cells from damage.

4. Improved immune function: Antioxidants can also help support immune function, which can be beneficial for overall health and recovery after exercise. Exercise can temporarily suppress the immune system, leaving the body vulnerable to infection and illness. Consuming antioxidant-rich foods can help support immune function and reduce the risk of illness.

Some examples of antioxidant-rich foods include berries, leafy greens, citrus fruits, nuts, seeds, and dark chocolate. By incorporating a variety of antioxidant-rich foods into your diet, you can help support your body's recovery after exercise and reduce inflammation, which can be beneficial for overall health and well-being.

G. The role of vitamins and minerals in supporting overall health and physical activity, including vitamin D, calcium, and iron.

Vitamins and minerals play a crucial role in supporting overall health and physical activity. Here are some key examples of how specific vitamins and minerals support physical activity:

1. Vitamin D: Vitamin D is important for bone health, as it helps the body absorb calcium. Adequate vitamin D intake is essential for supporting bone strength and reducing the risk of fractures. Vitamin D also plays a role in supporting immune function and reducing inflammation, which can be beneficial for overall health and recovery after exercise.

2. Calcium: Calcium is essential for bone health and is necessary for the body to build and maintain strong bones. Adequate calcium intake is especially important for individuals who

engage in weight-bearing activities such as walking, running, and weightlifting.

3. Iron: Iron is important for delivering oxygen to the muscles during physical activity, which can improve endurance and performance. Iron deficiency can lead to fatigue, weakness, and decreased athletic performance, so it's important to consume adequate amounts of iron through food or supplements.

4. Magnesium: Magnesium is essential for muscle and nerve function and can help reduce muscle cramping and soreness.

5. B vitamins: B vitamins play a role in energy metabolism and can help support energy levels during physical activity.

6. Potassium: Potassium is important for maintaining proper fluid balance and muscle function and can help reduce muscle cramping and soreness.

Incorporating a variety of nutrient-rich foods into your diet can help ensure that you are getting all the vitamins and minerals needed to support physical activity and overall health. Useful sources of these key vitamins and minerals include dairy products, leafy greens, nuts, seeds, whole grains, and lean proteins. Additionally, supplements may be necessary for individuals who have difficulty meeting their nutrient needs through diet alone. It's important to consult with a healthcare provider or registered dietitian to determine the appropriate supplement regimen for your individual needs.

What differentiates the benefits of vitamin D2 from those of vitamin D3?

Vitamin D2 (ergocalciferol) and vitamin D3 (cholecalciferol) are two forms of vitamin D, which is an essential nutrient for human health. While they are both forms of vitamin D, there are some differences between them in terms of sources, absorption, and benefits:

Sources:

Vitamin D2 (ergocalciferol) is derived from plant-based sources. It is often found in fortified foods like dairy products, orange juice, and cereals. It can also be obtained from supplements.

Vitamin D3 (cholecalciferol) is primarily derived from animal-based sources. It is synthesized in the skin when it is exposed to sunlight (UVB rays). It can also be found in fatty fish, egg yolks, and some fortified foods. Like D2, it is also available in supplement form.

Absorption:

Research indicates that vitamin D3 (cholecalciferol) is superior in elevating vitamin D levels in the bloodstream compared to vitamin D2 (ergocalciferol). This advantage stems from the stronger binding of vitamin D3 to receptors in the body, enhancing its absorption and utilization. Additionally, vitamin D3 exhibits a longer half-life within the body when contrasted with vitamin D2.

Benefits:

Both vitamin D2 and D3 are important for bone health as they help regulate calcium and phosphorus levels in the body, promoting bone mineralization and preventing conditions like rickets and osteoporosis.

Vitamin D plays a role in immune function, and cardiovascular health, and may have protective effects against certain cancers, although more research is needed to fully understand these benefits.

Some studies suggest that vitamin D3 may be more effective than D2 in reducing the risk of fractures and falls in older adults.

Supplementation:

Both vitamin D2 and D3 forms are available as supplements, but for individuals at risk of vitamin D deficiency, such as those with limited sun exposure, older adults, or individuals with certain medical conditions, vitamin D3 supplements are typically recommended due to their enhanced absorption and efficacy.

In summary, while both vitamin D2 and D3 are important forms of vitamin D and contribute to overall health, vitamin D3 (cholecalciferol) is more effective at raising vitamin D levels in the blood and is often the preferred form for supplementation. However, obtaining vitamin D through a combination of sunlight exposure and a balanced diet is also important for maintaining optimal levels of this essential nutrient.

H. Tips for eating on-the-go during long walks, including healthy snack options and portable meals.

1. Plan ahead: Before your walk, plan out your snacks and meals for the day. This will help ensure you have enough food to fuel your body and prevent hunger.

2. Pack portable snacks: Choose snacks that are easy to carry and don't require refrigeration, such as nuts, dried fruit, protein bars, and trail mix.

3. Bring fresh fruits and vegetables: Pack fresh fruits and vegetables that are easy to eat on-the-go, such as apples, bananas, baby carrots, and snap peas.

4. Don't forget protein: Protein is important for muscle repair and recovery after exercise. Pack protein-rich snacks, such as hard-boiled eggs, cheese sticks, and jerky.

5. Hydrate with water: Water is the best choice for staying hydrated during a long walk. Bring a refillable water bottle with you and drink regularly throughout the day.

6. Try coconut water: Coconut water is a natural source of electrolytes and can be a good alternative to sports drinks. Look for brands with no added sugars.

7. Pack a sandwich: Sandwiches are a great option for a portable, balanced meal. Choose whole grain bread and fillings such as turkey, avocado, and vegetables.

8. Make a salad in a jar: Layer your favorite salad ingredients in a mason jar for a portable, healthy meal. Choose a protein source, such as chicken or tofu, and pack the dressing separately.

9. Bring a thermos of soup: Soup can be a satisfying and warming meal during a long walk. Pack a thermos of soup, such as vegetable or lentil soup.

10. Stock up on healthy snacks at rest stops: If you're walking a long distance and need to stop for a break, look for healthy snack options at rest stops, such as fresh fruit or yogurt.

Overall, it's important to choose snacks and meals that are nutrient-dense and provide the fuel your body needs during a long walk. Plan ahead, pack portable snacks and meals, and stay hydrated with water and electrolyte-rich beverages.

11. Consider nutrient timing: It's important to time your meals and snacks appropriately to fuel your body before and during your walk. Aim to eat a balanced meal with carbohydrates, protein, and healthy fats about 2-3 hours before your walk. Then, eat a snack or small meal every 2-3 hours during your walk to keep your energy levels up.

12. Opt for low-glycemic index (GI) foods: Low-GI foods are digested more slowly and provide a sustained release of energy. Examples of low-GI foods include whole grain bread, oatmeal, sweet potatoes, and most fruits.

13. Avoid processed and sugary snacks: Processed snacks such as chips, crackers, and candy provide empty calories and can cause a crash in energy levels. Instead, choose whole, minimally processed foods that will provide sustained energy.

14. Be mindful of portion sizes: While it's important to fuel your body during a long walk, it's also important not to overeat. Pack snacks and meals in appropriate portion sizes to avoid feeling sluggish or uncomfortable.

15. Incorporate variety: Eating a variety of nutrient-dense foods will help ensure you get all the nutrients your body needs during a long walk. Mix up your snacks and meals with different fruits, vegetables, whole grains, proteins, and healthy fats.

By following these tips and selecting nutrient-rich foods, you can support your energy levels and overall health during long walks.

I. The benefits of meal planning and preparation to ensure that healthy food is readily available for an active lifestyle.

Meal planning and preparation can have a significant impact on an active lifestyle by ensuring that healthy food is readily available. Here are some benefits of meal planning and preparation:

1. Saves time: By planning and prepping meals in advance, you can save time during the week. This can be especially important

for busy individuals who don't have a lot of time to cook and prepare meals.

2. Reduces stress: Knowing what you're going to eat ahead of time can help reduce the stress of having to make decisions about food on a daily basis. This can also help you avoid the temptation of unhealthy fast food or convenience items.

3. Promotes healthy eating: By planning and preparing healthy meals, you can ensure that you're getting the nutrients you need to fuel an active lifestyle. This can help improve overall health and wellbeing, as well as support weight management goals.

4. Saves money: Eating out or buying convenience items can be expensive. Meal planning and preparation can help save money by allowing you to buy ingredients in bulk and cook meals at home.

5. Reduces food waste: When you plan your meals in advance, you're less likely to buy ingredients that will go to waste. This can help reduce food waste and save money on groceries.

Overall, meal planning and preparation can help you stay on track with your nutrition goals and support an active lifestyle. It can take some time and effort to get started, but the benefits are well worth it.

J. The importance of consulting a registered dietitian or nutritionist for personalized nutrition and hydration recommendations.

1. Personalized recommendations: A registered dietitian or nutritionist can provide personalized recommendations that are tailored to your individual needs, preferences, and health goals. They can consider factors such as your age, gender, activity level, and any medical conditions you may have.

2. Evidence-based advice: Registered dietitians and nutritionists are trained professionals who have a deep understanding of nutrition science. They can provide evidence-based advice that is based on the latest research and guidelines.

3. Safety: Consulting a registered dietitian or nutritionist can help ensure that you are consuming a safe and balanced diet that meets all of your nutritional needs.

They can also help identify any potential nutrient deficiencies or excesses and provide recommendations to address them.

4. Accountability: Working with a registered dietitian or nutritionist can help keep you accountable and motivated to make healthy choices. They can provide ongoing support and guidance as you work towards your nutrition and hydration goals.

5. Long-term success: By working with a registered dietitian or nutritionist, you can develop a personalized nutrition and hydration plan that is sustainable and tailored to your lifestyle. This can help ensure long-term success in achieving your health and fitness goals.

6. Disease prevention and management: Registered dietitians and nutritionists can provide guidance on how to prevent or manage various health conditions, such as diabetes, heart disease, and high blood pressure, through proper nutrition and hydration.

7. Sports nutrition: If you're an athlete or engage in regular physical activity, a

registered dietitian or nutritionist can provide guidance on how to optimize your nutrition and hydration for improved performance and recovery.

8. Weight management: If you're looking to lose weight or maintain a healthy weight, a registered dietitian or nutritionist can provide personalized guidance on how to achieve your goals through proper nutrition and hydration.

9. Food allergies and intolerances: If you have food allergies or intolerances, a registered dietitian or nutritionist can help ensure that you are consuming a safe and balanced diet that meets all of your nutritional needs.

10. Sustainability: Registered dietitians and nutritionists can provide guidance on how to make sustainable food choices that are good for both your health and the environment.

Overall, consulting a registered dietitian or nutritionist can be an important step in optimizing your nutrition and hydration for an active lifestyle. They can provide personalized recommendations, evidence-based advice, and ongoing support to help you achieve your goals.

Michael Luxiey: "Just as a car needs quality fuel to run smoothly, your body deserves the best nutrition for a walk that takes you places."

Chapter 10:
Walking Groups and Communities

1- Walking and Community
    a. Walking groups and clubs
    b. The benefits of joining these groups
    c. Tips for finding and joining a walking group

a. Walking groups and clubs

Many communities have organized walking groups or clubs that offer regular opportunities for socializing and exercise.

    1. Walking groups and clubs are organized communities of people who come together regularly to walk for exercise and socializing. These groups can be found in most communities and are often organized by local organizations such as community centers, schools, or health clubs.

    2. Joining a walking group or club can provide many benefits. For one, it's an excellent way to stay motivated and committed to a regular walking routine. Walking with a group can also make the experience more enjoyable and social, as you can meet new people and make friends.

3. Additionally, walking in a group can be a safer option than walking alone, especially if you are walking in unfamiliar areas or at night. Group walking can also provide an opportunity to explore new places, as many groups organize walks in local parks or trails.

4. Most walking groups and clubs welcome people of all ages and fitness levels. Some groups may have a specific focus, such as seniors, women, or families with young children, while others may be more general in nature.

5. To find a walking group or club in your area, you can check with your local community center or health club, search online, or ask friends and family for recommendations. Many groups also have social media pages or websites where you can learn more about their activities and events.

b. The benefits of joining these groups

Here are some key benefits that you can discuss when encouraging someone to join a walking group or club:

1. Motivation and Accountability: Joining a walking group or club provides motivation for sticking to a regular walking routine. When you know that others are counting on you to show up, it's easier to stay committed to your fitness goals.

2. Socializing: Walking in a group is an excellent way to meet new people and make friends. Walking with others can provide an opportunity to have conversations and share experiences, which can be beneficial for mental health and well-being.

3. Safety: Walking in a group can be a safer option than walking alone, especially if you are walking in unfamiliar areas or at night. In a group, you are less likely to be targeted by criminals, and you will have the support of others if you experience any issues.

4. Improved Health: Joining a group can be a fun and effective way to achieve health benefits such as improved cardiovascular health, strengthened muscles, and weight loss through walking, a low-impact exercise.

5. Access to New Places: Walking groups and clubs often organize walks in local parks, trails, and other areas that you may not have explored on your own. Joining a group provides an opportunity to discover new places and enjoy the outdoors.

By discussing these benefits, you can help someone understand why joining a walking group or club can be a great idea for their physical and mental well-being.

c. Tips for finding and joining a walking group.

1. Determine your fitness level: Before joining a walking group or club, it's essential to assess your fitness levels. Some groups may be geared towards more experienced walkers, while others may be designed for beginners. Make sure to choose a group that matches your fitness level.

2. Check for schedules and locations: Look for groups that meet at a time and location that is convenient for you. Consider how far you are willing to travel and what time of day you prefer to walk. You can also check the group's schedule to ensure it fits your schedule.

3. Research different groups: Take the time to research different walking groups and clubs in your area. Look online, check community bulletin boards, and ask around to find groups that match both your interests and needs.

4. Attend a few walks: Once you have identified a few groups that interest you, attend a few walks to get a feel for the group's dynamics

and whether it's a good fit for you. Most groups welcome new members and are happy to have you join them for a walk or two before deciding whether it's a good fit.

5. Communicate with group leaders: If you have any questions or concerns about joining a walking group or club, don't hesitate to reach out to the group leaders. They can provide you with more information and help you make an informed decision about whether the group is right for you.

By following these tips, you can find and join a walking group or club that suits your interests, fitness level, and schedule. Remember, walking in a group can be a fun and effective way to stay motivated and committed to your fitness goals, while also providing an opportunity to socialize and explore new places.

2- Virtual walking communities

a. The benefits of joining a virtual walking community

b. Virtual walking communities

a. The benefits of joining a virtual walking community.

Joining a virtual walking community can provide many benefits. Here are a few:

1. Convenience: One of the primary benefits of joining a virtual walking community is the convenience it provides. You can participate in the community from the comfort of your own home or office, and you can connect with others at any time that works for you.

2. Flexibility: Virtual walking communities are often more flexible than in-person groups. You can walk on your own schedule, choose your route, and participate in challenges or events that fit with your lifestyle.

3. Support and Motivation: Joining a virtual walking community can provide you with a support system of like-minded individuals who can motivate and encourage you on your fitness journey. Many virtual communities have online forums or social media groups where members can share tips, advice, and encouragement.

4. Accountability: Virtual walking communities can provide a sense of accountability to help you stay on track with your fitness goals. You can track your progress and

participate in challenges or events that hold you accountable to your walking habits.

5. Accessibility: Virtual walking communities can be more accessible than in-person groups, particularly for those facing mobility or transportation issues. You can participate from anywhere, regardless of your physical location.

By joining a virtual walking community, you can stay motivated and committed to your fitness goals while connecting with others who share your interests. It's an excellent way to stay active, even when you can't physically be with others in a group setting.

b. Virtual walking communities

Here's some more information about the virtual communities, forums, social media groups, and fitness apps that offer support and encouragement to walkers:

1. **Strava:** Strava is a popular fitness app that allows users to track their walks, runs, and other workouts using GPS. The app has a social component that allows users to connect with friends and join groups. Users can share their activities with the community and give and receive kudos for their efforts. Strava also has several walking-focused groups that offer support and encouragement to walkers, such as the

"Walking for Health" group and the "Walking Challenge" group.

2. **MapMyWalk:** MapMyWalk is another popular fitness app that allows users to track their walks using GPS. The app has a social component that includes challenges and groups focused on walking and other fitness activities. Users can connect with other walkers, share their progress, and receive encouragement from the community. MapMyWalk also offers personalized training plans and route planning tools to help walkers reach their fitness goals.

3. **WalkJogRun:** WalkJogRun is a website and app that allows users to map out their walking routes and connect with other walkers. The site has several walking-focused groups that offer support and encouragement to walkers, such as the "Walk at Home" group and the "Walk and Talk" group. Users can also search for walking routes in their local area, track their progress, and share their accomplishments with the community.

4. **MyFitnessPal:** MyFitnessPal is a popular fitness app that allows users to track their food and exercise. The app has a social component that includes groups focused on walking and other

fitness activities. Users can connect with other walkers, share their progress, and receive encouragement from the community. MyFitnessPal also offers personalized nutrition and exercise plans to help users achieve their fitness goals.

5. **Facebook Groups:** There are many Facebook groups dedicated to walking, including walking challenges, support groups, and groups focused on specific walking goals or interests. Users can connect with other walkers, share their progress, and receive encouragement from the community. Facebook groups can also be a wonderful way to find local walking groups or events in your area.

6. **Fitbit Community:** Fitbit is a popular fitness tracker that allows users to track their steps, distance, and other activity metrics. The Fitbit Community is an online forum where users can connect with other Fitbit users, share tips and advice, and participate in walking challenges.

7. **Walking Connection:** Walking Connection is a website and forum dedicated to walking and hiking. The site offers resources and advice for walkers, as well as a forum where users

can connect with other walkers, share their experiences, and ask for advice.

8. **Walk at Home:** Walk at Home is a website and community dedicated to indoor walking workouts. The site offers a variety of walking workouts that can be done at home, as well as a community forum where users can connect with other walkers and share their progress.

9. **Fit Bottomed Girls:** Fit Bottomed Girls is a website and community focused on fitness and wellness for women. The site has a dedicated walking section, as well as a community forum where users can connect with other walkers, share their progress, and receive support and encouragement.

10. **Walking for Health:** Walking for Health is a UK-based organization that promotes walking as a way to improve health and well-being. The organization offers resources and advice for walkers, as well as a community forum where users can connect with other walkers and share their experiences.

11. **Walk with a Doc:** Walk with a Doc is a program that encourages walking and physical

activity as a way to improve health. The program offers local walking events led by healthcare professionals, as well as a virtual community where users can connect with other walkers and receive support and encouragement.

12. **Walk BC:** Walk BC is a website and community focused on walking and hiking in British Columbia, Canada. The site offers resources and advice for walkers, as well as a community forum where users can connect with other walkers, share their experiences, and ask for advice.

13. **Walk Score:** Walk Score is a website and app that helps users find walkable neighborhoods and walking routes in their local area. The site also offers a community forum where users can connect with other walkers and share their experiences.

14. **Walk and Bike Mendocino:** Walk and Bike Mendocino is a California-based organization that promotes walking and biking as a way to improve health and reduce carbon emissions. The organization offers resources and advice for walkers and bikers, as well as a community forum where users can connect with

other walkers and bikers and share their experiences.

15. **Walking World:** Walking World is a UK-based website and community focused on walking and hiking. The site offers a variety of walking routes and trails, as well as a community forum where users can connect with other walkers, share their experiences, and ask for advice.

By joining one or more of these virtual communities, forums, social media groups, and fitness apps, walkers can connect with others who share their interests, receive support and encouragement, and stay motivated to reach their fitness goals.

3- Walking events and challenges

    a. The best walking events in the world
    b. Training schedules for these events
    c. Tips for participating in these events.
    d. Tips for participating in the Camino del Norte.
    e. Nutrition advice
    f. Tips for Staying Motivated

a. Walking Events and Challenges

There are many walking events and challenges around the world, each with their own unique features and attractions.

1. Camino de Santiago: This is a pilgrimage route that stretches across Spain and leads to the city of Santiago de Compostela, where the remains of Saint James are said to be buried. It's a popular walking route with many people undertaking it as a spiritual journey or for adventure. The route is about 500 miles long and typically takes about a month to complete.

The Camino del Norte, Spain: A 900 km pilgrimage route along the northern coast of Spain, passing through small fishing villages and historic cities.

2. The Inca Trail: This is a four-day trek through the Peruvian Andes to the ancient ruins of Machu Picchu. The trail is one of the most popular walking routes in the world and offers stunning scenery and historical sites.

The Inca Jungle Trail, Peru: A 4-day trek to Machu Picchu that includes hiking, biking, and ziplining through the jungle.

3. The Great Wall of China: This is a long-distance hike along one of the most iconic

structures in the world. The Great Wall of China stretches over 13,000 miles and offers a unique perspective on Chinese history and culture.

4.   The West Highland Way: This is a 96-mile walking route through the Scottish Highlands, starting in Milngavie and ending in Fort William. The route takes walkers through beautiful scenery, including lochs, mountains, and forests.

5.   The Appalachian Trail: This is a 2,200-mile walking route that stretches from Georgia to Maine in the United States. The trail is one of the most famous long-distance hikes in the world and offers a chance to experience the natural beauty of the eastern United States.

6.   The Australian Alps Walking Track: This is a 655 km long-distance walking track that passes through the high country of Victoria, New South Wales, and the Australian Capital Territory. The track offers stunning alpine scenery and the chance to see wildlife such as kangaroos, wallabies, and wombats.

7. Mount Kilimanjaro Trek: Trek to the highest peak in Africa and take in the stunning views of the surrounding landscapes.

8. The Lycian Way, Turkey: Walk through ancient ruins, rugged coastline, and high peaks on this 509 km trail.

9. Laugavegurinn Trail, Iceland: Explore the highlands of Iceland on this 55 km trek through colorful rhyolite mountains, hot springs, and glacial valleys.

10. The Haute Route, Switzerland/France: A 180 km trek through the Swiss and French Alps, passing through high mountain passes and offering breathtaking views.

11. The Tour du Mont Blanc: A 170 km trek around the Mont Blanc Massif, passing through France, Italy, and Switzerland.

12. The West Coast Trail, Canada: A 75 km trek along the west coast of Vancouver Island, through old-growth forests and rocky beaches.

13. The Milford Track, New Zealand: A 53 km trek through the Fiordland National Park, including views of the iconic Milford Sound.

14. The Overland Track, Australia: A 65 km trek through the Tasmanian wilderness, passing by Cradle Mountain and Lake St Clair.

15. The Coast to Coast Walk, England: A 309 km trek across England, from the Irish Sea to the North Sea.

16. The Great Ocean Walk, Australia: A 104 km trek along the rugged coastline of Victoria, featuring stunning ocean views and local wildlife.

17. The Chilkoot Trail, Canada/USA: A historic 53 km trek through the Klondike Gold Rush region, from Alaska to British Columbia.

18. The Kumano Kodo, Japan: A network of pilgrimage routes in Japan, passing through beautiful mountain scenery and ancient temples.

19. The Hebridean Way, Scotland: A 247 km trek along the west coast of Scotland, through remote islands and beautiful beaches.

20. The Cotswold Way, England: A 164 km trek through the rolling hills and picturesque villages of the Cotswolds.

21. The Abel Tasman Coast Track, New Zealand: A 60 km trek along the golden beaches and turquoise waters of Abel Tasman National Park.

22. The Jordan Trail, Jordan: A 650 km trek across Jordan, passing through historic sites and beautiful desert landscapes.

23. The Westweg Trail, Germany: A 285 km trek through the Black Forest region of Germany, with stunning views and charming villages.

24. The Dales Way, England: A 127 km trek through the Yorkshire Dales, passing through beautiful landscapes and charming towns.

25. The Kungsleden Trail, Sweden: A 440 km trek through the Swedish Lapland, featuring beautiful mountain landscapes and the chance to see the Northern Lights.

26. The Transcaucasian Trail, Armenia/Georgia: A 750 km trek through the Caucasus Mountains, featuring stunning mountain views and ancient cultural sites.

27. The Kalalau Trail, Hawaii, USA: An 18 km trek through the beautiful Na Pali Coast on the island of Kauai, featuring stunning ocean views and waterfalls.

b. Training schedules for the events and challenges

1. Marathon des Sables:

20-week training plan that includes running, walking, and strength training, gradually increasing mileage and endurance each week.

2. Appalachian Trail thru-hike:

6-month training plan that includes hiking, cross-training, and strength training, gradually building up to longer hikes and heavier backpacks.

3. Everest Base Camp trek:

12-week training plan that includes hiking, cardio exercise, and strength training, gradually building up to long hikes with elevation gain.

4. Tour du Mont Blanc:

16-week training plan that includes hiking, cardio exercise, and strength training, gradually building up to long hikes with elevation gain.

5. Camino de Santiago:

12-week training plan that includes walking, cross-training, and strength training, gradually building up to long walks with a backpack.

6. Mount Kilimanjaro trek:

12-week training plan that includes hiking, cardio exercise, and strength training, gradually building up to long hikes with elevation gain.

7. The Lycian Way, Turkey:

16-week training plan that includes hiking, cardio exercise, and strength training, gradually building up to longer hikes with elevation gain.

8. The Milford Track, New Zealand:

12-week training plan that includes hiking, cardio exercise, and strength training, gradually building up to long hikes with elevation gain.

9. The Inca Trail, Peru:

8-week training plan that includes hiking, cardio exercise, and strength training, gradually building up to long hikes with elevation gain.

10. The West Coast Trail, Canada:

16-week training plan that includes hiking, cardio exercise, and strength training, gradually building up to long hikes with elevation gain.

11. Ultra-Trail du Mont Blanc:

24-week training plan that includes running, hiking, and strength training, gradually increasing mileage and elevation gain each week.

12. The Haute Route:

16-week training plan that includes cycling, hiking, and strength training, gradually building up to long rides with elevation gain.

13. The Colorado Trail:

12-week training plan that includes hiking, cross-training, and strength training, gradually building up to longer hikes with elevation gain.

14. The West Highland Way, Scotland:

12-week training plan that includes hiking, cross-training, and strength training, gradually building up to longer hikes with elevation gain.

15. The Pacific Crest Trail:

6-month training plan that includes hiking, cross-training, and strength training, gradually building up to longer hikes with elevation gain.

16. The Great Himalaya Trail:

24-week training plan that includes hiking, cardio exercise, and strength training, gradually building up to long hikes with elevation gain.

17. The Snowman Trek, Bhutan:

24-week training plan that includes hiking, cardio exercise, and strength training, gradually building up to long hikes with elevation gain.

18. The Camino del Norte:

12-week training plan that includes walking, cross-training, and strength training, gradually building up to long walks with a backpack.

19. The South Downs Way, England:

12-week training plan that includes hiking, cross-training, and strength training, gradually building up to longer hikes with elevation gain.

20. The John Muir Trail:

12-week training plan that includes hiking, cross-training, and strength training, gradually building up to longer hikes with elevation gain.

21. The Annapurna Circuit, Nepal:

16-week training plan that includes hiking, cardio exercise, and strength training, gradually building up to long hikes with elevation gain.

c. Tips for participating in these events.
You can add some tips for participating in these events by following these steps:

1.   Identify the event or challenge you want to provide tips for.

2.   Consider your own experience or research tips from other sources.

3.   Write down your tips in a clear and concise manner.

4.   Make sure your tips are relevant to the event or challenge and will be helpful for participants.

5.   Check for accuracy and make sure the tips are up to date.

6.   Format your tips in a way that is easy to read and follow, such as bullet points or numbered lists.

7.   Include your tips along with the event or challenge description in your response.

d. Tips for participating in the Camino del Norte.

1.   Make sure you have comfortable and durable walking shoes, as you will be walking long distances each day.

2. Pack light and only bring essential items, as you will need to carry everything with you.

3. Take care of your feet and make sure to rest them regularly.

4. Stay hydrated by drinking plenty of water and carry a refillable water bottle with you.

5. Make sure to plan your route and accommodations in advance, as the Camino del Norte can be busy during peak season.

6. Be open to meeting new people and making new friends, as the Camino del Norte is a social experience.

7. Take your time and enjoy the journey, as the Camino del Norte is about more than just reaching the destination.

e. Nutrition advice

1. Stay hydrated: Drink plenty of water and electrolyte-rich beverages before, during, and after your walk to stay properly hydrated.

2. Eat a balanced diet: Make sure to include a variety of nutrient-dense foods in your diet, such as whole grains, fruits, vegetables, lean proteins, and healthy fats.

3. Fuel up before your walk: Eat a meal or snack with complex carbohydrates, such as whole grains or fruits, a few hours before your walk to provide your body with energy.

4. Pack snacks: Bring along high-energy, easy-to-digest snacks such as energy bars, trail mix, or fruit to keep you fueled during long walks.

5. Replenish after your walk: Eat a post-walk meal or snack that includes carbohydrates and protein to help replenish glycogen stores and repair muscle tissue.

6. Consider supplements: Some athletes may benefit from taking supplements such as iron, vitamin D, or omega-3 fatty acids, but it's important to talk to your doctor or a registered dietitian before starting any supplement regimen.

7. Don't try anything new on race day: Stick to foods and drinks that you know work well for you during training and avoid trying new foods or supplements on race day.

8. Listen to your body: Pay attention to how your body feels during training and make adjustments to your diet and hydration as needed. If you have any concerns about your nutrition or hydration, talk to a doctor or registered dietitian.

f. Tips for Staying Motivated

1. Set specific, achievable goals: Having a clear goal in mind can help you stay focused and motivated. Make sure your goals are realistic and achievable for your current fitness level.

2. Create a training plan: Develop a training plan that includes specific workouts and goals. This will help you stay on track and measure your progress.

3. Mix it up: Incorporate different types of walking workouts, such as intervals, hills, or speed work, to keep your routine interesting and challenging.

4. Find a walking partner or group: Joining a walking group or finding a walking partner can provide accountability and social support.

5. Reward yourself: Celebrate your accomplishments, no matter how small they may be. Treat yourself to a healthy snack or a massage after a long walk.

6. Track your progress: Keep a record of your workouts and progress to help you see how far you've come and stay motivated to keep going.

7. Visualize success: Picture yourself achieving your goals and imagine how it will feel when you reach them.

8. Focus on the benefits: Remind yourself of the many benefits of walking, such as improved cardiovascular health, stress relief, and weight management.

9. Stay positive: Don't get discouraged by setbacks or bad workouts. Focus on the positive and keep moving forward.

Remember, motivation can ebb and flow, so be patient with yourself and keep working towards your goals.

4- Walking tours and hikes

1. Walking tours and hikes are popular activities in many communities around the world. These tours and hikes are designed to showcase the unique history, culture, or natural beauty of a specific location.

Walking tours often take place in urban areas and are led by knowledgeable guides who provide insight into the history and culture of the area. Hikes, on the other hand, are typically outdoor adventures that take participants through scenic natural landscapes, such as forests, mountains, or coastal areas.

Some walking tours and hikes may focus on a particular theme or topic, such as food, art, or architecture. Others may highlight a specific historical event or period, such as a walking tour of a city's historic district or a hike along a trail used by early settlers.

2. Participating in walking tours and hikes can offer a variety of benefits. For one, these activities provide an excellent opportunity to learn about a new place and its culture, history, or natural environment. They also

offer a chance to connect with others who share similar interests and to make new friends.

Walking tours and hikes can also provide physical and mental health benefits. Walking is a low-impact form of exercise that can improve cardiovascular health, reduce stress, and boost mood. Hiking, in particular, is a great way to improve fitness, strength, and endurance while enjoying the outdoors.

3.To find and join local walking tours or hiking groups, start by researching online. Many communities have websites or social media pages that list upcoming events and activities, including walking tours and hikes. You can also check with local tourist boards, parks and recreation departments, or nature centers to find out about organized tours or groups in your area.

Another option is to join online communities or groups that share your interests in walking or hiking. Websites like Meetup.com, for example, allow you to search for local groups that organize walking tours or hikes. These groups often welcome new members and can provide a fun and supportive way to explore a new place or enjoy the outdoors.

5- Walking for a cause

Walking can also be a way to raise awareness or support for a particular cause, such as a disease or social issue.

    a. How walking can be used as a tool for advocacy

    b. tips for organizing a fundraising walk.

    c. tips for creating a walking challenge for a cause you care about

a. how walking can be used as a tool for advocacy:

1. Breast cancer walk: Walking to raise awareness and funds for breast cancer research and treatment.

2. Alzheimer's walk: Walking to raise awareness and funds for Alzheimer's disease research and support services.

3. AIDS walk: Walking to raise awareness and funds for HIV/AIDS research and support services.

4. Hunger walk: Walking to raise awareness and funds for local food banks and hunger relief organizations.

5. Suicide prevention walk: Walking to raise awareness and funds for suicide prevention and mental health support services.

6. Environmental walk: Walking to raise awareness and funds for environmental causes,

such as protecting endangered species or fighting climate change.

7. Domestic violence walk: Walking to raise awareness and funds for domestic violence prevention and support services.

8. Autism walk: Walking to raise awareness and funds for autism research and support services.

9. Animal welfare walk: Walking to raise awareness and funds for animal welfare causes, such as ending animal cruelty or promoting pet adoption.

10. LGBTQ+ pride walk: Walking to show support for LGBTQ+ rights and equality.

b. 10 tips for organizing a fundraising walk:

1. Choose a cause: Decide on a cause or organization that you want to support through the walk.

2. Set a goal: Determine how much money you want to raise and set a fundraising goal.

3. Find a location: Choose a location for the walk that is accessible and safe for participants.

4. Set a date: Select a date and time for the walk that works well for participants and is convenient for the community.

5. Recruit volunteers: Recruit volunteers to help with planning, logistics, and day-of activities.

6. Create a website: Build a website or online platform to promote the walk, register participants, and collect donations.

7. Promote the walk: Use social media, flyers, and other marketing materials to promote the walk and encourage participation.

8. Secure sponsors: Reach out to local businesses and organizations to secure sponsorships and donations.

9. Plan day-of activities: Plan activities and entertainment for participants on the day of the walk to create a festive and engaging atmosphere.

10. Follow up: After the walk, thank participants and donors and share the results of the fundraising effort.

c. 10 tips for creating a walking challenge for a cause you care about:

1. Choose a cause: Decide on a cause or organization that you want to support through the walking challenge.

2. Set a goal: Determine how many steps or miles you want participants to walk and set a fundraising goal.

3. Create a team: Recruit a team of participants to join the challenge and help spread the word.

4. Find a platform: Choose a platform for participants to track their steps or miles, such as a fitness tracker app or website.

5. Set a timeframe: Decide on a timeframe for the challenge, such as a week or a month.

6. Create a website: Build a website or online platform to promote the challenge, register participants, and collect donations.

7. Promote the challenge: Use social media, flyers, and other marketing materials to promote the challenge and encourage participation.

8. Set up fundraising tools: Enable fundraising tools on your website or platform so participants can collect donations from friends and family.

9. Provide support: Offer support and encouragement to participants throughout the challenge, such as through weekly check-ins or motivational messages.

10. Follow up: After the challenge, thank participants and donors and share the results of the fundraising effort.

6- Walking and mental health:

Walking with others can also have a positive impact on mental health, providing social connection and a sense of purpose.

Walking is not only good for physical health but also for mental health. Walking with others can have a positive impact on mental health by providing social connection and a sense of purpose. Walking in a group can help reduce feelings of loneliness and isolation, increase feelings of belonging and connectedness, and provide opportunities for social interaction and support. Walking in nature can also have additional benefits for mental health by reducing stress, anxiety, and depression, and increasing feelings of well-being and relaxation.

Benefits:

1. Walking in a group can provide social connection and a sense of purpose, which can improve mental health and reduce feelings of loneliness and isolation.

2. Walking in nature can reduce stress, anxiety, and depression, and increase feelings of well-being and relaxation.

3. Walking can also improve self-esteem and self-confidence, which can have a positive impact on mental health.

Tips for finding a walking group or community:

1.   Research local walking groups or clubs in your area. Many cities and towns have walking groups that meet regularly for group walks.

2.   Join a community fitness center or gym that offers group fitness classes or walking groups.

3.   Use social media to find walking groups or communities. Facebook, Meetup, and other social media platforms can be great resources for finding walking groups in your area.

4.   Consider volunteering for a walking or hiking event, such as a charity walk or trail cleanup. This can be a fantastic way to meet new people and get involved in your community.

5.   Reach out to friends, family, or coworkers who may be interested in walking together. Walking with others can be a great way to strengthen relationships and build social connections.

6.   Look for walking groups or communities that are supportive and welcoming. You want to find a group that is inclusive and welcoming of all members, regardless of their fitness level or walking experience.

Chapter 11:
Advanced Walking Techniques

1. Power Walking
2. Nordic Walking
3. Interval Walking
4. Infinity Walking or Figure-Eight Walking

Who was the inventor of these techniques?

The techniques of power walking, Nordic walking, and interval walking have evolved over time, and it's difficult to attribute their invention to any one person or group. However, here's some brief background on the development of these techniques:

1. Power Walking

Power walking is a type of aerobic exercise that has been popular for decades, especially in the United States. It has its roots in the "racewalking" sport, which involves walking at a fast pace while always maintaining contact with the ground. Power walking as a fitness activity has evolved from this sport and became popularized in the 1980s and 1990s as a low-impact alternative to running.

Power walking is a form of walking that is faster and more vigorous than traditional walking. It typically involves swinging your arms vigorously and taking longer strides. Power walking can be a great cardiovascular workout and can help you burn more calories than regular walking. It can also be a low-impact alternative to running.

What are the benefits of Power Walking?

Power walking is a form of exercise that involves walking at a brisk pace with exaggerated arm movements to increase the intensity of the workout. Here are some benefits of power walking:

1. Burns more calories: Power walking is more effective than traditional walking for burning calories, making it an excellent option for maintaining a healthy weight.

2. Improved cardiovascular health: Power walking is a cardiovascular exercise that can help improve heart and lung function.

3. Low impact: Because power walking is a low-impact form of exercise, it is easier on the joints than high-impact activities like running.

4. Increased muscle strength: Power walking engages the muscles of the legs, core, and upper body, making it a great way to build overall strength and endurance.

5. Improved balance and stability: Power walking can improve balance and stability, making it a good exercise for older adults or those with balance issues.

6. Reduced stress on the back: Power walking can help reduce stress on the back and improve

posture by engaging the muscles of the core and upper back.

7. Accessible: Power walking can be done in a variety of settings, including urban environments, parks, and hiking trails, making it accessible to people of all ages and fitness levels.

Overall, power walking is an effective and low-impact form of exercise that can help improve cardiovascular health, burn calories, and build strength and endurance. It is also accessible and can be done in a variety of settings, making it a great option for anyone looking to improve their fitness and overall well-being.

What are the 10 steps of Power Walking? Power walking is a form of walking that involves a brisk pace and arm movements to increase the intensity of the workout. Here are ten steps to help you get started with power walking:

1. Start with proper equipment: Wear comfortable shoes that provide good support and allow for proper movement. You may also want to wear clothing that is designed for exercise.

2. Begin with a warm-up: Start with a five-minute warm-up of low-intensity walking to prepare your muscles for exercise.

3. Establish good posture: Keep your head up, shoulders back and relaxed, and engage your core muscles.

4. Increase your speed: Walk at a brisk pace that is faster than your normal walking speed.

5. Swing your arms: Move your arms in a natural, comfortable rhythm to help increase your pace.

6. Take longer strides: Take longer strides than you would when walking at a normal pace to increase your pace and intensity.

7. Focus on your breathing: Breathe deeply and rhythmically to help increase your endurance and stamina.

8. Monitor your heart rate: Use a heart rate monitor to track your heart rate and ensure you are staying within a safe range.

9. Stay hydrated: Drink water before, during, and after your power walking workout to avoid dehydration.

10. Cool down and stretch: After your power walking workout, take time to cool down with low-intensity walking and stretch your muscles to prevent injury.

By following these steps, you can safely and effectively incorporate power walking into your exercise routine and enjoy the many health benefits it offers.

2. Nordic Walking

Nordic walking originated in Finland in the 1930s as a way for cross-country skiers to train in the off-season. The use of poles was found to provide a full-body workout and to be an effective way to maintain cardiovascular fitness. The technique was popularized in the 1990s and has since spread to many countries around the world.

Nordic walking is a type of walking that originated in Finland and involves using poles to engage the upper body muscles while walking. Nordic walking poles are like ski poles and are designed to help you increase your speed and endurance while walking. Nordic walking can provide a full-body workout and can be a great way to improve your cardiovascular fitness and build strength in your arms, shoulders, and core.

What are the Benefits of Nordic Walking?

Nordic walking is a low-impact form of exercise that involves walking with poles. Here are some of the benefits of Nordic walking:

1. Full-body workout: Nordic walking engages the muscles of the upper body, lower body, and core, making it a full-body workout that can help to build strength and increase endurance.

2. Low impact: Because Nordic walking is a low-impact form of exercise, it is easier on the joints than high-impact activities like running.

3. Increased calorie burn: Nordic walking burns more calories than traditional walking, making it an effective way to maintain a healthy weight.

4. Improved cardiovascular health: Nordic walking is a cardiovascular exercise that can help to improve heart and lung function.

5. Improved balance and stability: The use of poles in Nordic walking can improve balance and stability, making it a good exercise for older adults or those with balance issues.

6. Reduced stress on the back: Nordic walking can help to reduce stress on the back and improve posture by engaging the muscles of the core and upper back.

7. Accessibility: Nordic walking can be performed in a variety of settings, including urban environments, parks, and hiking trails, making it accessible to people of all ages and fitness levels.

Overall, Nordic walking is a great form of exercise that offers numerous health benefits and is an excellent way to improve fitness and overall well-being.

What are the 10 steps of Nordic walking?

1. Start with proper equipment: Nordic walking requires special poles that are designed to help propel you forward.

2. Stand upright with good posture: Keep your head up, shoulders relaxed, and arms at your sides.

3. Place the poles behind you: Place the poles behind you and angled toward the back.

4. Plant the poles in front of you: As you step forward with one foot, plant the pole opposite to that foot on the ground in front of you.

5. Push off with the poles: As you push off with the back foot, use the poles to help propel you forward.

6. Swing your arms: As you swing your arms forward, plant the opposite pole in front of you.

7.   Keep your arms straight: Your arms should be straight but not locked, and you should not grip the poles too tightly.

8. Stride out: Take long strides to increase your pace and efficiency.

9. Focus on your breathing: Nordic walking can help improve your breathing, so try to breathe deeply and rhythmically as you walk.

10. Cool down and stretch: After your walk, take time to cool down and stretch your muscles to avoid injury.

By following these 10 basic steps, you can learn how to Nordic walk safely and effectively. With practice, you can increase your speed and distance and enjoy the many benefits of this popular fitness activity.

3.Interval Walking
Interval training has been used by athletes for many years to improve their performance, but the specific technique of interval walking is a relatively new concept. It is a variation of interval training that is adapted for walking, and the specific approach may vary depending on the individual or trainer. Interval walking has become increasingly popular in recent

years as a way to maximize the benefits of walking while minimizing the time commitment.

Interval walking involves alternating periods of high-intensity walking with periods of rest or lower-intensity walking. For example, you might walk briskly for two minutes and then slow down to a leisurely pace for one minute before picking up the pace again. Interval walking can be a great way to improve your fitness level and burn more calories compared to traditional walking. It can also be a good option for those who find it difficult to sustain a high-intensity pace for an extended period of time.

What are the benefits of interval walking?

Interval walking is a form of exercise that involves alternating between periods of high-intensity walking and periods of lower intensity or rest. Here are some benefits of interval walking:

1. Burns more calories: Interval walking can burn more calories than traditional walking, making it an effective way to maintain a healthy weight.

2. Improved cardiovascular health: Interval walking is a cardiovascular exercise that can help to improve heart and lung function.

3. Increased endurance: Interval walking can improve endurance by gradually increasing the

length of the high-intensity intervals and decreasing the length of the low-intensity or rest periods.

4. Improved muscle strength: Interval walking can engage the muscles of the legs, core, and upper body, making it a great way to build overall strength and endurance.

5. Reduced boredom: Interval walking can be more interesting and less monotonous than traditional walking, as it involves changing the pace and intensity of the exercise.

6. Accessible: Interval walking can be done in a variety of settings, including urban environments, parks, and hiking trails, making it accessible to people of all ages and fitness levels.

Overall, interval walking is an effective form of exercise that can help to improve cardiovascular health, burn calories, build endurance and strength, and make exercise more interesting and engaging. It is also accessible and can be done in a variety of settings, making it a great option for anyone looking to improve their fitness and overall well-being.

What are the 10 steps of interval walking?

Interval walking is a form of exercise that involves alternating periods of high-intensity walking with periods of low-intensity or rest walking. Here are ten steps to help you get started with interval walking:

1. Start with a warm-up: Begin with a five-minute warm-up of low-intensity walking to get your muscles ready for exercise.

2. Choose your intervals: Decide on the length of time you will spend walking at high intensity and the length of time you will spend walking at low intensity or resting.

3. Start with shorter intervals: If you're new to interval walking, start with shorter intervals and gradually increase them as you build up your stamina.

4. Increase your speed: During the high-intensity intervals, increase your walking speed to a pace that makes you feel out of breath.

5. Use a timer: Use a timer or interval training app to keep track of your intervals and make sure you stick to your plan.

6. Listen to your body: If you start to feel overly fatigued or out of breath, slow down or take a break.

7. Hydrate: Be sure to stay hydrated by drinking plenty of water before, during, and after your interval walking sessions.

8. Cool down: After you complete your intervals, spend a few minutes cooling down with low-intensity walking.

9. Stretch: Take time to stretch your muscles after your interval walking session to help prevent injury and improve flexibility.

10. Increase your intervals gradually: As you become more comfortable with interval walking, gradually increase the length of your high-intensity intervals and reduce the length of your rest intervals.

By following these steps, you can safely and effectively incorporate interval walking into your exercise routine and gain the many benefits of this type of workout.

4. Figure-Eight Walking or Figure-Eight Walking

Walking in a figure-eight pattern, commonly referred to as "figure-eight walking," is a specific type of walking exercise that involves moving in the shape of the number eight. This movement can engage different muscles and add variety to your walking routine. Here's how you can perform a figure-eight walking exercise:

1. Choose a Location: Find a spacious area where you can walk without obstacles. This can be a park, a large room, or any open space.
2. Imagine an Eight: Visualize the shape of the number eight on the ground. It consists of two circles connected by a center point.
3. Walk the Figure Eight:
    a. Start at the center point of the eight.
    b. Walk forward to the top of the first circle.

  c. Curve around and walk to the bottom of the first circle.

  d. Cross over to the second circle and walk to the top of it.

  e. Curve around and walk to the bottom of the second circle.

  f. Continue this pattern, creating a continuous figure-eight motion.

4. Maintain Good Posture: Keep your back straight, shoulders relaxed, and engage your core muscles as you walk.

5. Coordinate Arm Movements: Swing your arms naturally to enhance the overall engagement of your upper body.

6. Start Slowly: Begin with a slow and controlled pace until you feel comfortable with the figure-eight walking pattern.

7. Increase Intensity: As you become more accustomed to the movement, you can increase your walking speed to make the exercise more challenging.

This type of walking can help improve coordination, balance, and flexibility. It also adds a fun and dynamic element to your regular walking routine. As always, pay attention to your body, and if you have any health concerns, consult with a healthcare professional before trying new exercises.

What are the benefits of Figure-Eight Walking?

Walking in an 8-shaped or figure-eight pattern can offer several benefits, both physical and mental. Here are some advantages of incorporating this type of walking into your exercise routine:

1. Improved Coordination: Walking in a figure-eight pattern engages different muscle groups and challenges your coordination skills, promoting better overall body control.

2. Enhanced Balance: The continuous change in direction and weight shifting while walking in a figure-eight pattern can help improve balance, which is particularly beneficial for older adults or individuals working on stability.

3. Increased Core Strength: The figure-eight walking motion requires core stabilization to maintain balance and control. Over time, this can contribute to improved core strength.

4. Joint Flexibility: The varied movements involved in walking in a figure-eight pattern can help enhance joint flexibility, especially in the hips and ankles.

5. Cardiovascular Exercise: While not as intense as some cardio workouts, figure-eight walking can still elevate your heart rate, contributing to cardiovascular fitness.

6. Engagement of Different Muscle Groups: Walking in a figure-eight engages not only the muscles typically involved in walking but also those responsible for lateral movements, providing a more comprehensive workout.

7. Variety and Fun: Incorporating different walking patterns adds variety to your routine, making exercise more enjoyable and reducing the risk of boredom.

8. Mind-Body Connection: The intentional movement in a figure-eight shape encourages mindfulness and a connection between your mind and body, promoting a more focused and meditative experience.

9. Low Impact: Figure-eight walking is generally a low-impact exercise, making it suitable for a wide range of fitness levels and putting less stress on joints compared to higher-impact activities.

10. Accessibility: You can perform figure-eight walking indoors or outdoors, depending on the available space, making it a convenient and accessible exercise option.

It's important to note that individual responses to exercise can vary, and the benefits may depend on factors such as fitness level, health conditions, and consistency in performing the exercise. As with any new exercise routine, it's advisable to start slowly and consult with a healthcare professional if you have any concerns or pre-existing health conditions.

Remember to approach any new exercise or walking technique with caution, especially if you have pre-existing health conditions. It's always a good idea to consult with a healthcare professional or fitness expert before adopting a new and potentially strenuous exercise regimen.

Here are some references and books on power walking, Nordic walking, and interval walking:

1. Power walking:
•   "The Power Walking Handbook: Expert Advice for Health and Fitness from A to Z" by Nina Barough
•   "The Complete Guide to Power Walking: Everything You Need to Know to Burn Fat, Reduce Stress and Improve Your Health and Well-Being" by Mark Fenton and Dave McGovern
•   "Power Walking: Burn Fat, Reenergize, and Reduce Stress with this Simple Low-Impact Exercise" by Maggie Spilner

2. Nordic walking:
•   "Nordic Walking: The Complete Guide to Health, Fitness, and Fun" by Claire Walter
•   "Nordic Walking for Total Fitness" by Suzanne Nottingham

- "Nordic Walking Step by Step: The Complete Guide" by Gill Stewart

3. Interval walking:

- "The Ultimate Guide to Interval Training: Maximize Your Workout with High-Intensity Interval Training (HIIT)" by Justin Roberts
- "Interval Walking for Weight Loss: How to Lose Weight Walking with These Interval Walking Workouts" by Dale L. Roberts
- "Interval Weight Loss for Life: The practical guide to reprogramming your body one interval at a time" by Nick Fuller

These books provide valuable information and insights on power walking, Nordic walking, and interval walking. Adding references like these can help lend credibility to your book and provide readers with additional resources to further explore these techniques.

Chapter 12:
Step by Step: Finding Inspiration and Motivation to Walk

1. Finding the Motivation to Start Walking When You Don't Feel Like It

2. Setting Realistic Goals for Your Walking Routine

3. Tips on How to Measure Progress and Track the Benefits of Walking

4. Making Walking a Social Activity: How to Connect with Others While Exercising

5. Incorporating Mindfulness into Your Walking Practice

6. Overcoming Obstacles to Consistent Walking: Time, Weather, and Other Challenges

7. Incorporating Strength and Stretching Exercises into Your Walking Routine

8. Keeping Your Walking Practice Interesting: Exploring New Routes and Techniques

9. Celebrating Your Success: How to Stay Motivated and Reward Yourself Along the Way

1. Finding the Motivation to Start Walking When You Don't Feel Like It

Starting a new habit like walking can be challenging, especially when you're not feeling motivated. However, there are several things you can do to find the motivation to start walking:

1.   Setting a goal: Setting a goal for yourself can help you stay motivated. For example, you could set a goal to walk for 30 minutes every day or to walk a certain number of steps each day.

2.   Finding a walking buddy: Having a friend or family member to walk with can help make the activity more enjoyable and hold you accountable.

3.   Making a playlist: Creating a playlist of your favorite songs or podcasts can make your walk more enjoyable and help distract you from any negative thoughts or feelings.

4. Starting small: If you're not used to walking, start with a small distance and gradually increase it over time. This can help prevent burnout and make the habit more sustainable.

5.   Focusing on the benefits: Remind yourself of the benefits of walking, such as improved mood, better cardiovascular health, and increased energy.

6.   Rewarding yourself: Set up a reward system for yourself, such as treating yourself to a favorite snack or activity after a certain number of walks.

7.   Choosing a time that works for you: Picking a time to walk that works for your schedule can help make it easier to stick to. If you're not a morning person, for example, it might be better for you to walk in the afternoon or evening.

8. Using a fitness tracker: Using a fitness tracker or pedometer can help you track your progress and motivate you to reach your goals. Seeing how many steps you've taken or how many calories you've burned can be a great source of motivation.

9.   Changing up your route: Walking the same route every day can get boring, so try changing up your route to keep things interesting. Explore new neighborhoods or parks or take a different path than you usually do.

10. Dressing for the weather: If you're not dressed appropriately for the weather, it can be harder to motivate yourself to go for a walk. Make sure you have comfortable shoes, appropriate clothing, and any necessary gear, like a raincoat or hat, to make your walk more comfortable.

11. Focusing on the present moment: Sometimes, we can get so caught up in our thoughts or worries that we forget to enjoy the

present moment. Focus on the sights, sounds, and sensations of your surroundings, and try to let go of any distracting thoughts.

12. Getting inspired: Reading about the benefits of walking, listening to podcasts or audiobooks about fitness and health, or watching inspiring videos or documentaries can help you stay motivated and focused on your goals.

Remember, the most important thing is to be consistent with your walking routine. Even if you don't feel motivated at first, sticking to your routine will help make walking a habit and part of your daily routine. Over time, you'll begin to see the benefits of walking and feel more motivated to continue.

2. Setting Realistic Goals for Your Walking Routine

Walking is a simple and effective way to improve your physical and mental health. Setting realistic goals for your walking routine can help you stay motivated and inspired to stick to your routine. Here are some tips to help you set realistic goals for your walking routine:

1. Starting small: It's important to start with a goal that's achievable and doesn't overwhelm you. If you're just starting out with a walking routine, try starting with a 10 or 15-minute walk

and gradually increase your time and distance. This will help you build your endurance and avoid injury.

2. Being specific: When setting goals for your walking routine, be specific about what you want to achieve. For example, you might set a goal to walk for 30 minutes each day, or to walk a certain number of steps per day. This will help you stay focused and motivated and give you a clear target to work towards.

3. Making it measurable: Use a pedometer, fitness tracker, or smartphone app to track your progress and measure your steps, distance, and time. This will help you track your progress and celebrate your achievements along the way.

4. Setting a deadline: Give yourself a deadline for achieving your walking goals. For example, you might aim to walk a 5K race in three months, which will give you a specific goal to work towards. Having a deadline can help you stay motivated and focused and give you a sense of urgency to achieve your goals.

5. Being realistic: When setting goals for your walking routine, be honest with yourself about your current fitness level and set goals that are

challenging but achievable. Don't set goals that are too difficult or unrealistic, as this can lead to frustration and disappointment.

6. Rewarding yourself: When you achieve your walking goals, be sure to reward yourself in some way. This could be something small, like treating yourself to a favorite snack or buying a new workout outfit, or something bigger, like taking a weekend trip or planning a spa day. Celebrating your achievements can help you stay motivated and feel good about your progress.

3. Tips on how to measure progress and track the benefits of walking include:

1. Set a daily step goal: Setting a daily step goal is a great way to stay motivated and track your progress. The American Heart Association recommends aiming for at least 10,000 steps a day, but you can adjust this goal based on your fitness level and personal preferences. Some people find that a higher step goal, such as 15,000 or 20,000 steps, is more challenging and helps them stay on track.

2. Keep a record of your steps: Recording the number of steps you take each day is a great way to track your progress and stay accountable. You can do this manually in a journal or use a tracking

app on your smartphone or fitness tracker. There are many different apps and devices available, so find one that works for you and stick with it.

3. Monitor your heart rate: Monitoring your heart rate during your walks can help you gauge the intensity of your workout and make adjustments as needed. Your heart rate should increase during exercise, but it shouldn't be too high or too low. Most fitness trackers will provide you with a target heart rate zone based on your age and fitness level.

4. Track your distance: Tracking the distance you walk can help you set goals and monitor your progress over time. Most fitness trackers will measure distance in miles or kilometers. You can also use online mapping tools, such as Google Maps, to plan your route and estimate your distance.

5. Pay attention to other metrics: Many fitness trackers also measure other metrics, such as calories burned, active minutes, and sleep quality. These metrics can provide valuable insights into your overall health and fitness. For example, tracking your sleep quality can help you identify patterns and make adjustments to improve your sleep hygiene.

6. Celebrate your progress: Celebrating your progress can help you stay motivated and engaged. When you reach a milestone, such as achieving your step goal for a week or walking a certain distance, take a moment to celebrate and acknowledge your achievement. This can be as simple as giving yourself a pat on the back or treating yourself to a small reward.

Remember, walking is just one part of an overall healthy lifestyle. To maximize the benefits of walking, be sure to also eat a balanced diet, get enough sleep, and engage in other forms of physical activity, such as strength training and stretching.

7. Vary your route: Walking the same route every day can get boring and make it harder to stay motivated. Varying your route can help keep things interesting and challenge your body in new ways. Try exploring new neighborhoods, parks, or trails to mix things up.

8. Increase your intensity: To get the most benefit from walking, you should aim to walk at a brisk pace that raises your heart rate. If you find that your walks are getting easier, try increasing your intensity by walking faster or incorporating

short bursts of jogging or running into your routine.

9. Set other goals: In addition to step and distance goals, you can also set other goals related to walking. For example, you could aim to walk for a certain amount of time each day or set a goal to climb a certain number of stairs or hills on your walks.

10. Join a walking group: Joining a walking group can be a great way to stay motivated and accountable. Look for local walking groups or join a virtual group online. You can also recruit friends or family members to walk with you on a regular basis.

11. Take breaks when needed: If you're new to walking or have a health condition that affects your mobility, it's important to listen to your body and take breaks as needed. Don't push yourself too hard and be sure to rest and hydrate when you need it.

12. Analyze your data: Many fitness trackers and apps provide detailed data on your walking habits, such as your average speed, step count, and heart rate. Take the time to analyze this data and look for patterns or areas where you can

improve. This can help you make adjustments to your routine and get more out of your walks.

Remember, the most important thing is to find a routine that works for you and stick with it. Walking regularly, even for just a few minutes a day, can have a big impact on your health and wellbeing.

4. Making Walking a Social Activity: How to Connect with Others While Exercising

Walking is a great way to exercise, and it can also be a social activity. Here are some tips on how to connect with others while walking and make it a fun and motivating experience:

1. Join a Walking Group: Joining a walking group is an excellent way to meet new people who share your interest in walking. You can join a local walking club, a hiking group, or a running group. Many cities have walking groups for seniors or groups that focus on walking for fitness. You can find these groups through local community centers, fitness centers, or online social media groups.

Walking with others can help you stay motivated, and you can also make new friends along the way. It's also an opportunity to share tips and advice with others who have similar interests. In a walking group, you can enjoy the benefits of walking while also having the added social component.

2. Walk with a Friend or Family Member: Walking with someone you know can be a great way to catch up and spend time together while getting some exercise. You can make it a regular activity by scheduling a weekly or monthly walking date. Walking with someone else can also help motivate you to stick to your routine and make it more enjoyable.

3. Participate in Charity Walks: Participating in charity walks is a great way to give back to your community while connecting with others who share your passion for walking. Many charity organizations organize walks and runs to raise money for a good cause, and you can join them as a team or as an individual.

The Charity walks can be an excellent opportunity to meet new people and socialize while doing something good for others. You can choose a cause that is close to your heart and raise money by asking for pledges from family and friends.

4. Use Social Media: Social media can be a great way to connect with other walkers and find new walking routes in your area. You can join walking groups on Facebook or follow walking-related hashtags on Instagram or Twitter to find other people who share your interests. You can also share your own walking photos or experiences to inspire others and start conversations.

5. Explore New Routes: Walking in the same area can get monotonous, so try to explore new routes with friends or family. You can also search for walking trails or hiking trails near you and explore them with a group. This can make your walking experience more enjoyable, and you can discover new places while exercising.

Exploring new routes can also provide an opportunity to connect with nature and enjoy the great outdoors. It's an excellent way to relieve stress, and it can be a fun way to bond with friends or family.

6. Volunteer for a Walking Event: Volunteering for a walking event, such as a charity walk or race, can be a great way to meet other walkers and feel like you're part of a larger community. You can help with registration, staffing water stations, or cheering on participants. Many events rely on volunteers, so it's easy to get involved.

7. Use Apps or Wearables: Using apps or wearables can be a fun way to connect with other users who share your goals. Many apps and wearables track your steps and connect you with other users who are also using the app. Some of these apps also have challenges and competitions that can motivate you to walk more and connect with others who share your goals.

For example, the app Strava allows you to track your walks and connect with other users in your area. You can also join challenges and compete with others to achieve your walking goals.

8. Walking Meetings: If you work in an office environment, you can suggest walking meetings instead of sitting in a conference room. Walking meetings can be

more productive, and they can also help you connect with your colleagues on a personal level.

Walking meetings can be a great way to break up the workday and get some exercise while also discussing work-related topics. It can also help to build relationships with colleagues outside of the workplace.

9. Organize Walking Events: Organizing a walking event can be a fun way to connect with others who enjoy walking. You can organize a walking event in your community, invite friends and family, and make it a social event. You can also include activities such as picnics or games to make it more enjoyable.

For example, you can organize a charity walk in your community and invite friends and family to participate. You can also organize a walking tour of your city and invite others to join you. It's an opportunity to socialize, get some exercise, and discover new places in your community.

In conclusion, walking can be a great social activity, and there are many ways to connect with others while exercising. Joining a walking group, participating in charity walks, exploring new routes, using apps or wearables, having walking meetings, and organizing walking events are some of the ways to make walking a fun and motivating experience.

5. Incorporating Mindfulness into Your Walking Practice

Walking can be a wonderful opportunity to incorporate mindfulness into your daily routine. It allows you to connect with your body, your surroundings, and your breath, and can be a powerful tool for reducing stress and increasing overall well-being. Here are some tips for incorporating mindfulness into your walking practice:

1. Start with Intention: Before beginning your walk, take a moment to set an intention for your practice. This can be a simple statement or phrase that reflects what you want to get out of your walk. For example, you might set an intention to focus on your breath, or to appreciate the beauty around you. By setting an intention, you are creating a sense of purpose for your walk and giving yourself a focus to return to if your mind begins to wander.

2. Pay Attention to Your Breath: As you walk, pay attention to your breath. Notice the rhythm and depth of your inhales and exhales. You might find it helpful to count your breaths or use a mantra to help focus your attention. If your mind begins to wander, gently bring your attention back to your breath. This can help to calm your mind and bring a sense of relaxation to your body.

3. Observe Your Surroundings: Take in the sights, sounds, and smells around you as you walk. Notice the colors of the trees and flowers, the chirping of birds, and the feel of the sun or wind on your skin. You might also pay attention to the texture of the ground beneath your feet or the sensation of your clothes against your skin. By being fully present in your environment, you can connect more deeply with the world around you.

4. Focus on Your Body: Tune in to your body as you walk. Notice the sensations in your feet, legs, and arms. Pay attention to your posture and alignment. You might also notice any areas of tension or discomfort and try to release them as you walk. By

bringing awareness to your body, you can become more grounded and centered.

5. Practice Gratitude: As you walk, take time to appreciate the simple things in life. Express gratitude for the beauty of nature, the warmth of the sun, or the company of a friend. You might also think about things in your life that you are grateful for, such as your health or your relationships. Focusing on gratitude can help shift your mindset to a more positive and peaceful place and can help you to feel more content and fulfilled.

Remember that mindfulness is a practice, and it takes time and effort to cultivate. Be patient with yourself and enjoy the journey. Walking mindfully can be a beautiful way to connect with yourself, your surroundings, and the present moment.

6. Overcoming Obstacles to Consistent Walking: Time, Weather, and Other Challenges

Walking is a wonderful form of exercise and can have numerous benefits for both physical and mental health. However, it can be challenging to maintain a consistent walking practice in the face of obstacles such as time constraints, inclement weather, or other challenges. Here are some tips for overcoming these obstacles and staying motivated to walk regularly:

1.   Make it a priority: One of the most important things you can do to maintain a consistent walking practice is to make it a priority in your life. This might mean scheduling your walks into your calendar, setting reminders on your phone, or finding a walking buddy who will help keep you accountable. You can also try setting goals for yourself, such as aiming to walk a certain number of steps or miles each week, to help keep you motivated and focused.

2.   Get creative with your schedule: If you're struggling to find time for walking, try getting creative with your schedule. For example, you might try walking during your lunch break or taking a walk after dinner. You can also break up your walking sessions into shorter intervals throughout the day if that works better for you. The key is to find a schedule that works for your lifestyle and to stick to it as consistently as possible.

3. Dress for the weather: Weather can be a major obstacle to walking, but with the right gear, you can walk comfortably in almost any conditions. Invest in appropriate clothing and footwear for the weather in your area and consider layering your clothing for added warmth or protection. You can also carry a small umbrella or rain poncho in case of unexpected rain. With the right gear, you can make walking a year-round activity.

4. Find a walking partner: Having a walking partner can be a great motivator and can make your walks more enjoyable. Consider joining a walking group in your community or recruiting a friend or family member to walk with you. You can also use social media or online communities to connect with other walkers and find accountability partners. By walking with someone else, you'll be more likely to stick to your routine and have fun in the process.

5. Mix it up: If you find yourself getting bored or losing motivation, try mixing up your walking routine. This might mean exploring new routes, incorporating interval training or other forms of exercise,

or listening to music or podcasts while you walk. By keeping things fresh and interesting, you can stay motivated and engaged with your walking practice. You might also consider setting yourself challenges, such as walking a certain number of steps in a day or trying to beat your personal best time on a particular route. Whatever you do, make sure to keep it fun and enjoyable so that you'll look forward to your walks each day.

Remember that consistency is key when it comes to building a habit of walking. By overcoming obstacles and staying motivated, you can make walking a regular part of your routine and enjoy the many benefits it has to offer.

7. Incorporating Strength and Stretching Exercises into Your Walking Routine

In addition to being a great form of cardiovascular exercise, walking can also be a great opportunity to incorporate strength and stretching exercises into your routine. By adding these exercises to your walking practice, you can increase your flexibility, balance, and overall fitness. Here are some tips for incorporating strength and stretching exercises into your walking routine:

1. Warm up: Before you begin your walk, take a few minutes to warm up your muscles. This can help to prevent injury and prepare your body for exercise. You might do some light stretching or walk at a slower pace for the first few minutes to get your body ready for activity.

2. Incorporate strength exercises: Walking is a great form of cardiovascular exercise, but it can also be an opportunity to incorporate strength exercises. Look for opportunities during your walk to add in strength exercises such as lunges, squats, or calf raises. You can also use a park bench or other sturdy surface for tricep dips, push-ups, or step-ups. By incorporating strength exercises into your walk, you can increase your overall fitness and build lean muscle mass.

3. Stretch after your walk: Once you've finished your walk, take a few minutes to stretch your muscles. This can help to increase your flexibility, reduce muscle soreness, and prevent injury. Focus on stretching the major muscle groups in your legs, back, and shoulders, holding each stretch for 10-30 seconds. Some great

stretches to include are calf stretches, hamstring stretches, and quadricep stretches.

4. Use walking as a warm-up or cool-down: Walking can also be a great warm-up or cool-down activity for other forms of exercise. For example, you might start your workout with a brisk walk to get your heart rate up and prepare your muscles for exercise or end your workout with a slower walk to help bring your heart rate back down and prevent injury.

5. Mix it up: To keep things interesting and challenging, try mixing up your strength and stretching exercises. You might alternate between different exercises during your walk or try different stretches after each walk. You can also change the intensity or duration of your exercises to make them more challenging. By keeping your routine fresh and varied, you'll be more likely to stick with it and see results.

Remember, incorporating strength and stretching exercises into your walking routine can be a fantastic way to increase your overall fitness and improve your health. By being intentional and creative with your exercises, you can make the most of your walking practice and enjoy all the benefits it has to offer.

8. Keeping Your Walking Practice Interesting: Exploring New Routes and Techniques

Walking is a simple yet effective way to stay active, reduce stress, and improve overall health. However, even the most dedicated walkers can get bored with the same routine and scenery. To keep your walking practice interesting, you can explore new routes and techniques. Here are some ideas to help you stay motivated and inspired:

1. Explore new areas: Walking the same route every day can get monotonous, so try to explore new areas whenever you can. You might discover new parks, scenic routes, or neighborhoods that you enjoy. Try walking in different areas during separate times of day to see how the scenery changes.

2. Use a GPS app: GPS apps like Strava or MapMyWalk can help you track your route, distance, and speed. They also have features that allow you to discover new paths and trails in your area, which can help keep your walking practice interesting. You

can also use these apps to set goals and track your progress.

3. Walk with a friend: Walking with a friend is a wonderful way to stay motivated and make the experience more enjoyable. You can chat and catch up while getting some exercise, and you might even discover new routes together. If you don't have a walking buddy, try joining a walking group in your area.

4. Try different walking techniques: Walking doesn't have to be a monotonous activity. There are several walking techniques that you can try to switch things up. For example, power walking involves taking faster, longer strides, while Nordic walking involves using poles to engage your upper body muscles. You can also try interval walking, where you alternate between walking at a moderate pace and walking at a faster pace.

5. Listen to music or podcasts: If you're walking alone, listening to music or podcasts can help pass the time and keep you entertained. You can create a playlist of your favorite songs or find podcasts that

interest you. You might even discover the latest music or learn something new while you walk.

6. Set goals and challenges: Setting goals and challenges can help keep you motivated and focused. For example, you could set a goal to walk a certain distance or time each week, or challenge yourself to walk up a steep hill or stairs. You can also set rewards for yourself when you reach your goals, such as buying a new pair of walking shoes or treating yourself to a massage.

Remember, the key to keeping your walking practice interesting is to mix things up and try new things. By exploring new routes, using GPS apps, walking with a friend, trying different techniques, listening to music or podcasts, and setting goals and challenges, you can keep your walking practice fresh and enjoyable.

9. Celebrating Your Success: How to Stay Motivated and Reward Yourself Along the Way

Achieving success can be a long and challenging journey, and it's essential to stay motivated and reward yourself along the way to maintain your drive and enthusiasm. Here are some tips on how to celebrate your success, stay motivated, and inspire yourself to achieve your goals:

1.   Set Achievable Goals: One of the most important things you can do when working towards a goal is to set achievable goals. Setting realistic and attainable goals helps you avoid frustration and discouragement that can come with setting goals that are too ambitious or unrealistic. Break down your goals into smaller, more manageable tasks, and set a deadline for each task. This way, you can track your progress and celebrate each milestone you reach.

2. Celebrate Small Wins: Celebrating small wins is a powerful motivator. It's easy to get discouraged when you're focused on the big picture, and it feels like you're not making progress. However, celebrating small wins along the way gives you a sense of accomplishment and helps you stay motivated. Celebrate each milestone you reach, whether it's finishing a task, hitting a sales target, or learning a new skill.

3. Keep a Record of Your Accomplishments: Keeping a record of your

accomplishments is a great way to stay motivated and inspired. You can create a journal or a digital document to keep track of your progress, milestones, and successes. This record can help you reflect on how far you've come, remind you of your accomplishments, and keep you motivated to keep going.

4. Find Inspiration from Others: Finding inspiration from others who have achieved similar goals is a terrific way to stay motivated. You can read books, listen to podcasts, or attend events where you can learn from others who have succeeded in areas that interest you. Surrounding yourself with people who motivate and inspire you can also help you stay motivated and inspired.

5. Take Time for Yourself: Taking time for yourself is essential to staying motivated and avoiding burnout. It's easy to get so caught up in pursuing your goals that you forget to take care of yourself. Schedule time each day or week to do something that makes you happy, whether it's reading a book, going for a walk, or spending time with friends and family. This will help you

recharge your batteries and come back to your work refreshed and motivated.

6. Treat Yourself: Treating yourself when you reach milestones is a fantastic way to celebrate your success and stay motivated. Rewards don't have to be expensive or extravagant. They can be as simple as your favorite meal, a relaxing bath, or a movie night with friends. The key is to recognize your accomplishments and give yourself a pat on the back for your hard work.

In conclusion, celebrating your success, staying motivated, and rewarding yourself along the way is crucial to achieving your goals. Keep setting achievable goals, celebrate small wins, keep a record of your accomplishments, find inspiration from others, take time for yourself, and treat yourself when you reach milestones. With these tips, you'll stay motivated and inspired to achieve your dreams.

Chapter 13:
Walking Tall: Posture, Safety, and Tips for Every Age and Ability

1. What is the Best Time of Day to Walk or Exercise?

A lot of people ask this question: what is the best time for a walk, morning or evening? Scientific research on lung function, temperature levels, and body rhythms suggests that it would be best if you walk around 6 p.m. However, walking in the morning also comes with great benefits for improving the body's overall metabolic rate.

A. Morning Walk or Exercise:

If you are an early riser, morning workouts will fit into your schedule. However, night owls may struggle with an early fitness session.

Pros:

For early risers, morning workouts fit into the schedule.

Morning walks provide a feeling of physical energy for hours.

Air pollution levels are lowest in the morning.

Consistent exercise in the morning helps establish a routine.

Cooler temperatures in summer facilitate outdoor exercise.

Fewer distractions in the morning.

You can gain time for exercise by starting your day earlier.

The body adjusts to your exercise time, so if you're training for a morning walk event, train in the morning.

B. Lunchtime Exercise:

Many people break up their workday with healthy activities. However, some may find it inconvenient to change in and out of workout clothes.

Pros:

A brisk walk significantly improves blood flow to the brain, making you sharper in the afternoon.

Stress relief from work, school, and home stresses.

Body temperature levels are higher than in the morning.

Exercise helps regulate appetite, potentially curbing break-time snacking.

Exercise during lunch may make the workout feel easier.

C. Late Afternoon Exercise:

If you have free time in the late afternoon, it would be a brilliant idea to schedule exercise. However, this schedule doesn't work for everyone.

Pros:

Afternoon exercise helps regulate food intake for dinner.

Body temperature peaks around 6 p.m.

Muscles are warm and flexible, reducing the risk of injury.

Perceived exertion is lowest in the afternoon.

Excellent for stress relief after a day.

D. Evening Exercise:

Here's the best time to schedule your evening walking session. Before starting, consider these benefits:

Pros:

Helps curb nighttime snacking.

Ideal for connecting with family after dinner while engaging in healthy activity.

Muscles are warm and flexible in the evening.

Perceived exertion is low.

You can work out harder and faster.

2. Walking for Weight Loss:

In recent years, staying active and walking have become trendy. Achieving a specific daily step count has significantly improved daily physical activity levels. Physical activity is better than none.

If you're aiming to manage your weight, walking can be one of the best tools. Here are some tips if you're looking to shed extra pounds through walking.

Duration of Daily Walks for Weight Loss

To lose weight, some health experts and diet programs recommend brisk walking.

- ❖ Aim for 30 to 90 minutes of brisk walking approximately five times a week.
- ❖ You can vary your walking time from day to day.
- ❖ Total weekly walking time should be at least 150 minutes.
- ❖ Walk fast enough to reach a moderate exercise zone (60-70 percent of maximum heart rate).
- ❖ Break up walking time into periods of 10 minutes or longer.
- ❖ Walking briskly for longer than 30 minutes at a time can enhance the fat-burning process after warming up.

Consistency is key for burning calories and improving metabolism to establish new habits. On non-walking days, consider incorporating strength training exercises.

Once you've achieved your weight loss goal and are working to maintain it, engage in 60 to 90 minutes of moderate-intensity physical activity. Avoid consuming more calories than you expend throughout the day.

Walking for Weight Loss TIPS

> **Check the weather.**

The last thing you want is to get caught in a rainstorm in the middle of your walk. It's important to check the weather forecast in the morning to determine the best time for a walk. If you plan to walk around 5 p.m., but the weather forecast predicts rain, it would be best to reschedule your walk for lunchtime. Moreover, it is recommended to carry a charged phone with you in case the weather takes a turn; there might be a need for someone to pick you up.

> **Hydrate**

If you are heading out for a long walk, make sure that you are hydrated. Always stay hydrated throughout the day. It is recommended to drink two cups of water 30-60 minutes before your walk so it's out of your system. When you return from the walk, make sure to drink a glass of water to rehydrate yourself. Moreover, it would be best to avoid all types of sugary sodas and electrolyte drinks. If you are walking at moderate intensity, water is enough to rehydrate your body.

- **Get the right gear.**
Toss away the old flip-flops, and it's the best time to get a new pair of sneakers. It will help you a lot with posture during the walk and also reduce the risk of injury. If you have a suitable pair of sneakers on, it will make your walking a longer distance more comfortable.

- **Focus on Form**
Walking itself does not require skill and is very natural. However, some posture and form cues can help enhance the walk. It would be best if you focused on keeping your chin up and shoulders square. Activate your core and keep your back straight. Engage your glutes with each step, and focus on tucking your buttocks inward for optimal posture.

- **Pick up the Pace!**
Walking in intervals is considered the best way to burn more calories and make your walk enjoyable. However, in terms of walking, there

are three different types of paces. The first one is a stroll, similar to window shopping, about a 3/4 difficulty on a scale of 10. Then comes a brisk walk, in which you make an effort, about a 4/5 difficulty. Finally, there is a power walk, where you are on a mission, about a 5/6 difficulty.

Warm up with a stroll. After that, aim for a brisk pace throughout the walk and push to a power walk pace every five minutes to get your heart rate up. Pay attention to the duration you can maintain a power walk pace and aim to increase it gradually each time. It is fascinating to know that power walking for weight loss makes a huge difference in your overall health.

➢ **Set a Goal**
If you want to optimize your walking pace, aim for 1.5 miles per 30 minutes or 3 miles per hour. This is a brisk pace of 20 minutes per mile. If you cannot commit to walking for an hour or 30 minutes, then anything is better than nothing and contributes to your daily step count tremendously.

➢ **Walk on an Incline**
If you are indoors, a treadmill allows you to manipulate your incline. This plays an essential role in enhancing the caloric burn of your walk.

On the flip side, if you are outside, try to opt for a hilly area to optimize your walk. It is essential to consider that increasing incline enhances the workout's intensity and reduces the impact on your legs and joints.

3. What If You Can't Walk for 30 Minutes?

Life can be busy. However, if your schedule doesn't permit you to walk continuously for 30 minutes, there is a way to break it up into walking two or three times daily for shorter periods of 10 minutes at a brisk pace.

It is fascinating to know that walking counts as exercise nearly any way you do it. It would be helpful to designate the primary purpose beforehand. If you are mainly looking to unplug, leave the technology at home and push the pace.

> ### ➤ How to Get Started
>
> Experts suggest that adults should get at least 150 minutes of moderate-intensity aerobic activity weekly. It can be broken down into small and doable spurts of exercise. If you want walking as an aerobic activity of choice, here's how to get started. To get started walking, you only need a suitable pair of walking shoes. It would be best to call a friend or

family member to walk with you. You can also add walking into your daily routine with some ideas like:

- If you commute, get off the bus one stop early and walk the rest of the way.
- Park farther away from your office than usual.
- Consider walking instead of driving while you run errands. Consider completing your tasks while incorporating exercise at the same time.

> **Check with the Doctor Before Starting**

It is especially essential if you are suffering from any medical or orthopedic conditions. Such conditions can limit your walking ability. No doubt, walking is the best exercise to help patients with diabetes and high blood pressure but ensure that your doctor knows the activities you do so that they can advise you accordingly.

If someone is suffering from hip, knee, ankle, or foot issues, it can limit their walking ability. Consulting a sports medicine doctor is recommended to determine safe exercises for individuals with these issues. A sports medicine doctor can provide an appropriate exercise prescription, minimizing the risk of injuries as they start their fitness journey.

➢ **Keep Safety in Mind**
Finding a safe route for a walk is also important. You must be careful, depending on the area you are walking in, and be conscious of your surroundings. Don't crank up the playlist so loudly that you can't hear the vehicles and pedestrians around you. Along with this, make sure to wear reflective clothing if you are walking early in the morning or late at night.

➢ **Start Slow and Progress Slowly**
Starting slowly is advisable, as it allows you to gauge your current fitness level. If you can only walk for a certain number of minutes, you have your baseline. Even if it is for five or 10 minutes at a time, that's enough. From there, gradually pick up the pace.

As your fitness level improves, you will start to notice, and you are allowed to walk rapidly at a set distance in a short time. It builds the endurance to walk longer than the last time.

> **Make it a Habit.**
> For beginners, it is recommended to take a walk after a meal. You are already in the habit of eating breakfast, lunch, as well as dinner. You can start with walking for 10 minutes after each meal. However, you can start doing it after just one meal if you notice that this strategy does not fit your schedule.

> **Remember to warm up.**
> Warming up your muscles is always good before exercise. Walking is a form of warming up. There are a few options here. You can start extra slowly, giving the body a few minutes or so to wake up or get the blood flowing to the muscles that need it. After that, you can pick up the pace as you see fit.

To warm up your body for a walk, you can do some upper body shoulder rolls, swing your legs in place, roll your foot from heel to toe, do body squats, and rotate your torso left and right.

> **Stretch afterward if you can!**
> Stretching your lower-body muscles, hamstrings, and calves just after a walk is essential. Keep in mind that stretching after walking helps improve blood circulation, so the muscles can heal and decrease the stiffness that can happen after a workout. Holding and pushing for at least 30 seconds maximizes its effects.
>
> While it seems reasonable to do some stretches after a walk when you can, it's not mandatory every time. If some days you have time for a quick walk, that's fine. The body and mind will be better for it.

4. What About Your Posture?

While walking, it is crucial to practice good posture. Keep in mind that walking may cause injuries to the feet or back. Stand tall, tuck your abs in, and keep your lower back from arching as you walk. Begin with quick and small steps to start your program, and as you progress, increase both the length of your steps and your pace. In terms of posture, bend your arms at the elbow and place your hands in the center of your body. Keeping your elbows fixed in this position makes it easier to swing your arms as you walk, giving your upper body the exercise it needs along with your legs.

Furthermore, push yourself along with your back foot while walking. As you lift

your feet, show the sole of your back foot. Ensure you wear well-fitting shoes and maintain correct posture. Set your fitness goals, make a plan, and enjoy walking your way to fitness.

➤ **Safety Suggestions While Walking**
Walking is the safest way to exercise, but you should still look out for unexpected hazards.

1. See a doctor for a proper check-up before starting a new fitness program. This is especially crucial if you are aged over 40 years, overweight, or haven't exercised in a long time.

2. Always choose walks that suit your age and fitness level. Warm-up and cool down with a slow walk to ease in and out of the exercise session.

3. Wear loose and comfortable clothing and appropriate footwear to avoid blisters or shin splints.

4. Bring waterproof clothing to stay dry in case of rain.

5. Carry an umbrella to fend off unleashed and unfriendly dogs.

6. Before bushwalking, check the weather forecast and take all the appropriate safety measures.

7. Look out for hazards in alpine/coastal areas.

8. Drink plenty of water before and after the walk. However, if you are taking a long walk, carry water with you.

➢ **Walking Tips for Children**

Statistics show that children are living more sedentary lives. Suggestions for encouraging a child to enjoy walking include:

1. If you notice that your child finds television and computer games more enjoyable than exercise, consider getting them a dog. The child's desire to love the animal can encourage him or her to take it on walks. However, keep in mind that dogs are not permitted in many national parks or other conservation reserves.

2. Boost your child's interest in outdoor activities.

3. Encourage the child's interest in nature through books and websites. In this way, they can discover their favorite animals and plants for themselves.

4. Schedule a regular family walk to build healthy habits for your children and spend time together.

5. While walking with children, ensure that the route and length of time spent walking are appropriate. A rule of thumb is approximately 1km per birthday.

6. Start good habits by taking young babies for walks in their pram. As they get older, encourage them to walk part of the way.

7. Look for self-guided nature walks that have been set up in many parks.

➢ **Walking Tips for Seniors**

Regular weight-bearing exercise improves cardiovascular fitness, bone strength, reduces excess body fat, and boosts muscle power. Walking is the best exercise for the elderly as it is low impact and high in health benefits. Here are some suggestions:

1. See a doctor for a proper check-up before starting any fitness program, especially if you are overweight or haven't exercised in a long time.

2. Pre-exercise screening is also useful for identifying individuals with medical conditions that may increase their risk of health problems during physical activity.

3. You can join a walking club that caters to your needs and age group.

4. Start your own walking club with friends and neighbors.

> **Walking Tips for People with Disabilities**

People with disabilities can also benefit from regular exercise. Here are some suggestions:

1. See a doctor for a medical check-up.

2. Some parks offer exclusive access, such as wheelchair access or other facilities.

3. Some sports clubs also offer sporting and recreational programs for people with disabilities of all ages.

4. A non-disabled person can help someone with a disability enjoy neighborhood walks or bushwalks.

5. Guide dogs are allowed in national parks, but domestic dogs, cats, or other pets are strictly forbidden.

Chapter 14:
"Walking Wonders: Real-Life Success Stories in Health Transformation"

1. John's Journey to Overcoming Obesity: A Tale of Resilience and Transformation

For years, John grappled with the burden of obesity, which not only affected his physical well-being but also cast a shadow on his self-esteem. Nevertheless, on an ordinary day, a spark of determination ignited within him. It kindled a remarkable transformation that would rewrite the story of his life.

Embracing a simple yet profound decision, John embarked on a modest yet unwavering commitment: a daily 30-minute walk. This initial endeavor was far from easy – each step was a poignant reminder of the challenge he faced, leaving him breathless after mere minutes. Yet, with remarkable persistence, he pressed forward, each footfall becoming a testament to his unyielding spirit. Over time, John's dedication bore fruit, his endurance growing until he could confidently stride for an hour or more without pause.

To amplify his newfound resolve, John enlisted the aid of a trusty fitness tracker, a companion that faithfully documented his daily steps and progress. Armed with data that showcased his incremental achievements, he discovered a wellspring of motivation previously untapped. He set ambitious goals for himself, eagerly embracing the opportunity to surpass them with each passing day. As his physical activity surged, so too did his commitment to nourishing his body. The siren call of junk food grew faint as John prioritized the vibrancy of fruits and vegetables, steering his diet toward a healthier course.

Months unfurled like pages in a transformative narrative, and John's dedication yielded astonishing results. The scale bore witness to a remarkable departure of over fifty pounds, but the transformation extended far beyond mere numbers. Medical markers of his well-being painted a compelling portrait of improvement: blood pressure readings that trended downwards and cholesterol levels that retreated from the precipice of concern. Yet, these quantitative triumphs were merely echoes of a far deeper shift. John's stride radiated newfound vitality; his confidence illuminated like a beacon.

What had once been a challenging endeavor had now woven itself into the very fabric of John's existence. Walking, once a daunting task, had become a ritual of solace and empowerment. The path to overcoming obesity, arduous as it was, had become an odyssey marked by triumph over adversity, willpower over temptation, and transformation over stagnation. John's story was no longer one of struggle but of resilience, no longer defined by the shadow of obesity *but illuminated by the radiance of his achievement. With each step, he walked not only toward better health but also toward a future imbued with the promise of possibility.*

2. Oprah's Story: Managing High Blood Pressure

Oprah had always been active, but she was diagnosed with high blood pressure during a routine checkup. Her doctor advised her to make lifestyle changes to manage her condition, and she decided to start by incorporating walking into her daily routine. However, she quickly discovered that it was a fantastic way to relieve stress and clear her mind.

She would wake up early every morning and go for a brisk 30-minute walk before work, and then take another 30-minute walk in the evening. She also started taking the stairs instead of the elevator and walking to nearby places instead of driving.

As Oprah became more consistent with her walking, she started to see improvements in her blood pressure readings. Her doctor was pleased with her progress and encouraged her to continue with her walking routine.

Over time, walking became a regular part of Oprah's daily routine. She would often take short walks throughout the day to break up her work and get some fresh air. She also started to make other healthy lifestyle changes, such as eating a more balanced diet and getting more sleep. Oprah's blood pressure stabilized, and she felt more energetic and focused than ever before.

3. Liam's Story: Overcoming Diabetes

Liam had been diagnosed with type 2 diabetes and was struggling to manage it with m. edication and lifestyle changes. He had tried various diets and exercise programs, but he always found them difficult to stick to. Then he decided to try walking. He would go for a 30-minute walk after each meal, as this had been shown to help regulate blood sugar levels.

At first, Liam found it challenging to find time for walking and to stay motivated. But he soon discovered that it was a fantastic way to clear his mind and relieve stress. He also started taking short walks throughout the day, such as during his lunch break or after work.

As Liam became more consistent with his walking routine, he started to notice improvements in his blood sugar levels. He also lost weight and felt more energized. With the support of his doctor, he was eventually able to reduce his medication and control his diabetes through diet and exercise alone.

Walking had become a powerful tool in managing Liam's diabetes and improving his overall health. He continued to make walking a regular part of his daily routine and found that it helped him stay focused and energized.

Liam was born in New York City, a bustling metropolis known for its iconic skyline and vibrant culture. One of his favorite places for walking was, Central Park. Nestled in the heart of Manhattan, Central Park offered a welcome respite from the city's hustle and bustle.

The park's sprawling 843 acres were a haven of natural beauty, with meandering pathways that led to hidden ponds, enchanting bridges, and peaceful meadows. Towering trees provided a canopy of shade, offering solace from the sun's rays during hot summer days.

One of Liam's cherished spots in Central Park was the Bethesda Terrace and Fountain. The grand terrace overlooked the picturesque Lake, and the intricate carvings and mosaics were a testament to the park's rich history and architectural beauty.

As the seasons changed, so did the landscape of Central Park. With the changing seasons came a transformation in the landscape of Central Park.

Cherry blossoms adorned the paths in spring, while vibrant foliage painted a tapestry of reds, oranges, and yellows in the fall. Even in the winter, when a blanket of snow covered the ground, Central Park transformed into a serene wonderland.

Liam's walks in Central Park became a source of inspiration and renewal. The park's tranquil atmosphere provided a perfect backdrop for his journey towards better health. With every step he took along the winding paths, he felt a sense of connection to nature and a profound gratitude for the healing power of walking.

4. Walking for Mental Health: Inspiring Stories

Footsteps to Resilience: Noah's Journey through Miami's Natural Parks

For years, Noah battled the relentless grip of depression, a persistent shadow that seemed impervious to the various attempts he made to free himself from its clutches. Despite undergoing therapies, testing various medications, and exploring a spectrum of treatments, his journey to recovery remained frustratingly elusive. The weight of isolation and hopelessness bore down on him, a seemingly impenetrable darkness that enveloped his existence.

Then, a transformative decision rippled through Noah's life one day, as he resolved to embark on a journey of healing through the simple act of walking. Breaking through the inertia that had kept him confined within the walls of his home, he took that crucial initial step, setting foot on a path that would lead him out of his cocoon of despair. His walks began modestly, threading through the familiar streets of his neighborhood. Gradually, they unfurled into explorations of the verdant parks and winding trails that crisscrossed his city of Miami.

One of Noah's favorite places to walk was in the sprawling expanse of the Everglades National Park, where the vibrant flora and diverse wildlife provided a serene backdrop to his thoughts. Another cherished spot was the Oleta River State Park, with its mangrove forests and winding waterways that offered a sense of solace and tranquility.

It was during these walks that Noah's friend Pipo became an indispensable companion. It was during these walks, that Noah's friend Pipo became an indispensable companion. Pipo's infectious energy and unwavering support provided a vital pillar of strength for Noah. Together, they would navigate the meandering trails, sharing stories and laughter, and finding solace in the beauty of nature.

In the nascent stages, the impact of these walks appeared subtle, their effect on Noah's profound depression seemingly imperceptible. The yoke of his emotional burden still lay heavy upon him, and motivation often wavered like a fragile flame in the wind. Yet, as the days stretched into weeks and the miles accumulated under his footsteps, an unexpected transformation started to unfold. The rhythmic cadence of his strides became a balm for his mind, a means to dispel the cacophony of negative thoughts and tether him to the ephemeral beauty of the present moment. With each footfall, a glimmer of positivity pierced through the shroud of darkness, kindling a spark of hope for a brighter future.

Gradually, the tempest within Noah's mind began to subside, as the practice of walking became an anchor of stability in the tumult of his emotions. A newfound resilience emerged, enabling him to confront life's challenges with a more composed spirit and navigate setbacks with greater equanimity. The cumulative effect of his walks infused his days with a renewed sense of purpose, granting him a lease on life that he had thought unattainable. While not a panacea for his mental health struggles, the simple act of walking had become a cornerstone of his well-being, illuminating a path from the depths of despair towards a horizon of possibilities.

5. In the realm of perpetual unease, Sarah had long been shackled by the chains of anxiety.

Each day was a battle, a constant struggle against overwhelming waves of stress that threatened to drown her spirit. The weight of her worries and fears seemed insurmountable, and she yearned for a respite from the relentless turmoil within her mind. It was in this tumultuous sea of emotions that a beacon of hope emerged, urging her towards a transformative journey.

One fateful day, a kindred soul reached out to Sarah, offering a lifeline to serenity. "Why not embark on a morning odyssey through the untamed landscapes of possibility?" her friend proposed, a glimmer of excitement dancing in their eyes. "A simple stroll to greet the dawn, a communion with the world before the day's clamor ensues."

Initially met with skepticism, Sarah hesitated at the threshold of change. The notion of breaking free from her cocoon of apprehension was daunting, an audacious leap into the unknown. Yet, a flicker of curiosity ignited within her. Tired of the ceaseless battle, she took the plunge, summoning her resolve to venture into the quietude of the early morn.

With the first rays of sunlight as her guide, Sarah embarked on her inaugural voyage through the cobwebbed alleyways of her neighborhood. As her footfalls resounded against the pavement, her thoughts were an orchestra of disquiet, the chorus of her anxiety crescendoing. But she pressed on, determined to confront her inner tempest head-on.

Then, as if orchestrated by fate itself, a metamorphosis began to unfold. As Sarah strode forth, an alchemical process ignited within her being. The crisp embrace of dawn's gentle breath intertwined with her own, dissolving the tendrils of unease that had ensnared her for so long. Nature's symphony played a soothing melody that harmonized with the rhythm of her heart.

With each step, a revelation dawned upon Sarah—a transformation of perspective, a shift in focus. The mundane became marvelous, the ordinary extraordinary. The world, once overshadowed by her anxiety, emerged as an oasis of wonder. The delicate petals of a rose, kissed by morning dew, whispered secrets of resilience. The steadfast oak tree, rooted in the earth's embrace, embodied unwavering strength.

Sarah's walks evolved into a ritual of renewal, an elixir for her weary soul. What began as a tentative journey had blossomed into a lifeline, threading vitality into her existence. The morning rambles became a sanctuary of self-discovery, a haven where anxieties were traded for revelations and apprehensions for aspirations.

As days turned into weeks, Sarah's metamorphosis was tangible. The tendrils of anxiety that once ensnared her began to loosen their grip. She found herself equipped with newfound tools—clarity in the face of chaos, and resilience amid uncertainty. Her once cacophonous inner landscape had transformed into a symphony of equilibrium.

It would be an exaggeration to say that the walks eradicated Sarah's anxiety entirely, for such an accomplishment is the stuff of legends. Yet, they had rewired her relationship with her fears, granting her dominion over her thoughts and emotions. No longer was she a helpless bystander; she had become the architect of her own narrative.

And so, in the luminous embrace of each morning's dawn, Sarah found herself anew. A triumphant phoenix rising from the ashes of apprehension, she soared on the wings of self-discovery. The walks had become her compass, guiding her towards a newfound sense of self-assuredness—a testament to the power of a single step towards the unknown, a testament to the potency of resilience in the face of adversity.

6. In the relentless whirlwind of workaday chaos, Tom had long been ensnared by the clutches of unyielding stress.

For years, he had battled against the ceaseless barrage of demands that his job hurled at him, his spirit weathered and his energy sapped. But one pivotal day, a spark of defiance ignited within him—a resolve to break free from the suffocating grip of his professional turmoil.

With a determination that burned like a meteor streaking across the sky, Tom embarked on a radical endeavor to reclaim his sanity. Armed with a newfound commitment to his well-being, he hatched a simple yet revolutionary plan: short walks during his lunch break. The very notion of extracting himself from the relentless grind was liberating, a declaration of independence from the all-encompassing clutches of his office walls.

And so, when noon's golden sun spilled its brilliance upon the urban landscape, Tom would don his metaphorical armor—a pair of well-worn sneakers— and march into battle against his own exhaustion. The rhythm of his steps synchronized with the cadence of his breathing, as if orchestrating a symphony of rejuvenation. The cacophony of deadlines and emails yielded to the melodious chirping of birds and the gentle rustle of leaves.

Initially, the siren song of his unfinished tasks lured him back to his desk like a sailor entranced by mermaids. Yet, he stood firm, allowing the world beyond his cubicle to envelop him. The streets became his sanctuary, the asphalt his canvas of solace. As he traversed the city blocks, his senses awakened to a kaleidoscope of urban vitality—the aroma of street food, the laughter of children, the vivacious colors of storefronts.

With each stride, Tom's transformation gained momentum. His soul drank deeply from the wellspring of nature's tranquility, his mind clearing like mist dissipating under the sun's fervent gaze. The worries that had once been his relentless companions began to retreat, cowed by the fortitude of his resolve. A newfound energy surged within him, a phoenix reborn from the ashes of his daily toil.

The walks, once a mere interlude, evolved into a vibrant ritual, a pilgrimage to a realm where stress bowed before the majesty of the present moment. Tom's return to the office was no longer a reluctant surrender; it was an exuberant revival, a rekindling of his spirit's fire. The shackles of exhaustion were shattered, replaced by a contagious vitality that colored his interactions, his decisions, and his very existence.

As days stretched into weeks and weeks into months, Tom's metamorphosis ripened, its impact radiating far beyond the sphere of his workplace. His colleagues noticed the transformation, mirroring his renewed enthusiasm and resilience. His infectious energy became an elixir, invigorating those around him, and his simple lunchtime escapades ignited a movement of self-care that swept through the office corridors.

Tom's journey, an odyssey of self-reclamation, had not only revolutionized his personal life but had cast ripples of change across his entire ecosystem. His stress was no longer a formidable foe; it had been tamed by his unwavering determination and his devotion to a daily ritual that had transformed into an act of liberation.

In the grand tapestry of existence, Tom's story stood as a testament to the power of one individual's resolve to challenge the status quo, to shatter the chains of routine, and to embrace the healing embrace of nature's embrace. And as he continued to stride forward, a modern-day hero of his own narrative, he left a trail of inspiration and revitalization in his wake—a beacon of hope for all who dared to seize the reins of their own well-being and embark on a journey towards a life untethered by stress.

Joyful Walks: Testimonials of Daily Exercise
7. Lila's Story: Walking for Fun and Fitness

Lila was always someone who struggled to find a form of exercise that she enjoyed. She tried running, yoga, and even weightlifting, but nothing really clicked for her. She would start off with enthusiasm, but after a few weeks, she would lose interest and give up.

One day, a friend suggested that she try walking for exercise. At first, Lila was skeptical. Walking seemed too simple and easy to be a real workout. But her friend insisted that walking was a great way to get fit, burn calories, and improve overall health. So, Lila decided to try it.

At first, she started small, taking short walks around her neighborhood. But soon, she found that she actually enjoyed walking. It was a chance to get some fresh air, clear her mind, and connect with her surroundings. She started walking for longer periods of time, exploring different paths and trails in her area.

Before she knew it, Lila was walking for 30 minutes a day, every day. She felt more energized, more focused, and more motivated than she had in years. And the best part was that she didn't have to make any major changes to her daily routine. She simply incorporated walking into her day, whether it was walking to work or taking a stroll after dinner.

As Lila continued to walk regularly, she noticed that her fitness level was improving. She was able to walk faster and farther without getting tired. She also noticed that she was losing weight and feeling stronger overall.

But even more than the physical benefits, Lila loved the mental and emotional benefits of walking. She felt happier, more relaxed, and more connected to nature. Walking had become a form of self-care for her, a way to take care of her body and mind.

Now, Lila can't imagine her life without walking. She's become an avid walker, exploring new trails and paths wherever she goes. And she encourages others to try walking for exercise, too. For Lila, walking isn't just a form of exercise, it's a way of life.

Title: "A Journey of Renewal: Unleashing Vitality Through the Power of Every Step"

8. Michael's Story: A Quest for Joyful Wellness and Vibrant Living

Michael's life was once shadowed by the weight of his health struggles and the looming threat of potential ailments. The shackles of excess weight and high blood pressure kept him from fully embracing the joys of life.

Frustration and disappointment clouded his attempts to regain control over his well-being. Little did he know that a simple, yet potent change would ignite a transformative journey, infusing his existence with electrifying energy.

In the heart of a neighborhood humming with the rhythm of daily life, Michael stood at a crossroads, uncertain yet resolute. His doctor's unconventional prescription echoed in his mind – an invitation to embark on a new path, one where each step held the promise of vitality and renewal. Walking, once a mere stroll in Michael's perception, now shimmered as a beacon of hope, an avenue to reclaim his health and rediscover the magic of life's simple pleasures.

As the sun's golden embrace bathed his surroundings, Michael tentatively set forth on his voyage of renewal. The pavement beneath his feet seemed to pulse with anticipation, a connection to a grander purpose. He took those initial steps, a blend of skepticism and determination propelling him forward. Each footfall was a proclamation of his commitment, a defiance against the inertia that had held him captive.

The first days were a symphony of effort and exhaustion. Glistening beads of sweat mirrored his resilience, marking his progress through the streets he had once overlooked. Yet, perseverance became his guiding star. The more he walked, the stronger he became. Breathlessness transformed into a steady rhythm, and fatigue metamorphosed into a persistent vigor. Michael's body, once reluctant, now thrived on the electrifying dance of movement.

Michael's walks evolved into a canvas of exploration, each route an opportunity to unravel the mysteries of his neighborhood. He ventured into lush parks, where trees whispered secrets and fragrant blooms painted the air with hues of serenity. Urban trails revealed hidden corners of his city, inviting him to forge an intimate connection with its beating heart. Every step was a brushstroke, crafting a vibrant tapestry of discovery and adventure.

Time became an ally as Michael's journey unfolded. With each passing week, his commitment deepened, and his walks grew longer. The clock's hands applauded his progress, pushing him to outpace his previous limits. The 20-minute challenge had transformed into 30, and then 40, a testament to his unwavering spirit. His transformation was nothing short of spectacular, the weight melting away like a cocoon yielding to a newly emerged butterfly.

The results were profound and undeniable. Michael's reflection radiated a newfound vibrancy, his skin aglow with the blush of revitalized health. The grip of high blood pressure loosened its hold, a silent victory etched in each beat of his heart. His story was no longer one of struggle, but of triumph over adversity. The scales tipped in favor of joy, and laughter became the anthem of his existence.

Raindrops became a melody, and sunshine a constant companion, as Michael's walks became a daily ritual, an enchanting rhythm that synchronized with the pulse of life. The world outside mirrored his inner transformation – vibrant, alive, and pulsating with energy. The mundane had morphed into the extraordinary, and each step propelled him forward, further away from his old self and closer to an exhilarating future.

Today, Michael stands as a testament to the boundless potential that lies within us all. His metamorphosis from a reluctant walker to a vibrant embodiment of well-being stands as a beacon of inspiration. With each step, he reaffirms the power of choice, the potency of commitment, and the electrifying energy that surges when we dare to embrace life's simple wonders.

In the mosaic of his journey, Michael found not just better health, but an exhilarating symphony of laughter, joy, and vibrant living. The page that was once blank is now adorned with the strokes of his resilience, the shades of his determination, and the brilliance of his transformation. With every leap from the mundane to the extraordinary, Michael's story now resides not just on the pages, but within the very fabric of his being – an electrifying testament to the limitless potential of the human spirit.

9. Leonardo's Story: Walking for Social Connection

Leonardo had always been an active person, but he found that most of his hobbies were solo activities. He wanted to find a way to be active and social at the same time. One day, he decided to try walking with a group.

At first, Leonardo was nervous about walking with others. He wasn't sure if he would be able to keep up or if he would fit in. But he decided to give it a try, and he found that walking with a group was a lot of fun.

He found walking with a group to be a lot of fun. He met new people, made friends, and had interesting conversations along the way. Walking had become a social activity for him, a way to connect with others while staying active.

Now, Leonardo walks with his group several times a week. He's found that walking with others has added a new dimension to his life. And he encourages others who are looking for a fun and social way to stay active to try walking with a group.

As Leonardo continued to walk with his group, he discovered that the benefits of social connection went beyond just having an enjoyable time. He found that walking with others helped him to stay accountable to his exercise routine, as he knew that his fellow walkers were counting on him to show up. This accountability helped him to stay motivated and committed to his fitness goals.

Leonardo also noticed that walking with others helped him to explore his community in new ways. His group would often take different routes or visit new parks or neighborhoods, which helped him to discover recent places that he might not have found on his own. He found that walking with others not only provided a sense of social connection but also helped him to feel more connected to his community as a whole.

In addition to the social and community benefits, Leonardo also found that walking with a group was a great way to improve his mental health. He often found himself feeling more relaxed and at ease after a walk with his group, as the physical activity and social interaction helped to reduce his stress and anxiety.

As Leonardo continued to walk with his group, he began to think about how he could encourage others to experience the benefits of walking for social connection. He started talking to friends and family members about his experiences and even organized a walking group at his workplace. He found that many people were interested in the idea but had been hesitant to try it on their own.

Through his efforts, Leonardo helped to create a community of walkers who not only stayed active but also formed meaningful social connections. Walking had become a way for people to come together, support each other, and explore their community in new and exciting ways. And it all started with Leonardo's decision to try walking with a group.

Weight Loss Triumphs: Sustained by Regular Walking

10. In the vibrant heart of bustling New York City, *a tale of transformation unfolds, centered around the resolute spirit of Angelina, a woman in her late twenties. Her struggle with weight had woven a veil of despair, ensnaring her in the relentless cycle of diets and exercises that yielded little. Yet, fate had a different path in store.*

On a serendipitous day, as Angelina strolled through the sprawling expanse of Central Park, laughter and vitality caught her attention. A group of fervent walkers powered through, their camaraderie infectious. Angelina hesitated only for a moment before stepping forward, her hesitance melting in the warmth of their welcome.

With every brisk step, a metamorphosis began to unfold. The pounds began to melt away, and the vitality she had longed for surged through her veins. Walking with a group became a source of immense joy and motivation for Angelina. She found that walking with others not only helped her lose weight but also enriched her life in numerous ways.

As Angelina immersed herself in the world of walking, she uncovered a tapestry of hidden gems within the city. Each park became a chapter in her story, each path a new adventure waiting to be explored. From the sun-dappled trails of Central Park to the tranquil embrace of the Charles River Esplanade in Boston, Angelina's footsteps traced a map of her triumphs.

Amidst the rhythmic cadence of her walks, destiny beckoned anew. Along the Charles River Esplanade, Angelina's path intersected with Mike's, a fellow seeker of solace and strength. United by their shared passion, their companionship kindled a bond that fortified their journeys. Together, they ventured forth, not only as friends but as kindred spirits on a shared pilgrimage.

Their strides became a symphony of determination, the echoes of their footfalls resonating with shared dreams and aspirations. As Angelina and Mike walked side by side, they wove a tapestry of support and encouragement, challenging each other to surmount obstacles and reach new heights. Their synergy sparked a blaze of motivation, igniting an unquenchable fire within.

Seasons turned, but Angelina and Mike remained unwavering in their dedication. Their victories were not fleeting; they etched their achievements into the annals of their lives. Weight loss was not a mere destination; it was the gateway to a realm of limitless possibilities. They scaled mountains of self-doubt and forded rivers of temptation, emerging stronger and more resilient with each conquest.

Years later, as they looked back upon their odyssey, Angelina and Mike stood as beacons of inspiration. Their narrative was no longer confined to the realm of personal achievement; it had transcended into a saga of shared triumph. Their footsteps had imprinted a legacy, inviting others to join the march toward a revitalized existence.

In a world often inundated with quick fixes and fleeting trends, the tale of Angelina and Mike resonates as a testament to the enduring power of steadfast commitment. Their narrative is a melody of renaissance, orchestrating a harmonious blend of determination and camaraderie. Through the simple act of walking, they unearthed a treasure trove of resilience, painting their lives with strokes of newfound vigor and vitality.

Dear reader, let the electrifying vigor of Angelina and Mike's journey be an anthem that reverberates within your soul. Embrace the transformative magic of each step, for within the rhythm of your own journey lies the symphony of renewal, waiting to be composed. The revitalization you seek is not a distant horizon; it is woven into the very fabric of your existence, awaiting only the resonance of your determination to awaken it.

Heart Health Victories: Achieved through Walking

11. In the heart of London, we meet Emily, *a tenacious 54-year-old who once stood at the precipice of health challenges. High blood pressure cast a looming shadow, a harbinger of potential heart disease. Yet, a consultation with her physician breathed hope into her world, illuminating the path of lifestyle amendments. Amidst the intricate dance of* *bustling urban life, Emily embarked on a journey of renewal through regular walks.*

Emily's tale, much like the pulse of a city, pulses with determination. A symphony of responsibilities once intertwined with her every breath, leaving scant room for self-care. A routine medical encounter marked the catalyst for her odyssey, unraveling the startling revelation of her vulnerability. Armed with a prescription for change, Emily endeavored to sculpt a new reality, interweaving physicality into her quotidian tapestry.

Stepping into her destiny, Emily navigated the labyrinthine streets of her existence, opting for stairs over elevators, strides over commutes. Lunch breaks metamorphosed into saunters of self-discovery, and evenings echoed with the rhythm of her footfalls. The embrace of each step was a nod to empowerment, a testament to her resolve to reclaim vitality.

As the weeks waltzed by, Emily's narrative painted a portrait of metamorphosis. The alchemy of walking ignited a cascade of benefits, each step echoing a harmonious symphony of health. The cacophony of stress, once a relentless percussion, waned, harmonizing her blood pressure. Her heart, akin to a phoenix, felt the caress of rejuvenation, the threat of heart disease dissipating like morning mist.

Emily's journey was a tapestry woven not only of physical vitality but also of emotional resilience. As her devotion to walking deepened, she observed the canvas of her life undergoing a spellbinding transformation. The weight of yesteryears diminished, blood pressure descended like a soft whisper, and vigor surged as if from an ancient wellspring. Her chronicles of arthritic tribulations were gradually supplanted by the cadence of her empowered footsteps.

Today, Emily stands as a testament to the narrative of triumph etched into the pavement of London's parks and avenues. A dedicated pilgrim in the temple of wellness, she navigates the urban tapestry with an invigorated zeal. Each park, each verdant sanctuary, serves as a testament to her rekindled spirit. Emily's odyssey, a breathtaking crescendo, reveals the symphony that emerges when the human spirit and the city's heartbeat align.

In this epoch of her existence, Emily has embraced the mantle of the walker. Her days now etched with an ineffable rhythm, she explores the city's soul, a voyage of perpetual discovery. Emily's journey through time and terrain mirrors the essence of metamorphosis, her footsteps an anthem to vitality reclaimed. Her saga resounds as a testament to the transformative power *of the humble walk, to the urbanite's odyssey to health, and to the resonance of a life well-lived.*

Nature's Embrace: Walking Stories of Discovery

12. Italy: "A Walk to Discover Hidden Treasures."

Francesco had always been proud of his city, Florence, known for its stunning art and architecture, delicious food, and rich history. As a native Florentine, he had spent his whole life exploring the famous landmarks and tourist hotspots. But one day, he realized that there was so much more to discover beyond the well-trodden paths. So, he embarked on a journey to explore the hidden treasures of Florence through walking.

With a map in hand and a spirit of adventure, Francesco set out to explore the Oltrarno district, located on the other side of the Arno River. He wandered through the narrow streets, where local artisans worked on their crafts, and came across the Santo Spirito Church, which houses works by famous Renaissance artists such as Filippo Lippi and Botticelli. After admiring the church's stunning interior, Francesco climbed up the Piazzale Michelangelo hill to enjoy panoramic views of the city from a unique perspective.

Feeling invigorated by his first discovery, Francesco continued his journey to the San Niccolò district, which lies hidden behind the medieval city walls. As he walked along the cobblestone streets, he stumbled upon the Torre Della Zecca, a historic tower that offers breathtaking views of the city from its top. Francesco climbed the narrow staircase to the tower's summit, where he gazed out at the city's iconic red roofs, the lush greenery of the Boboli Gardens, and the rolling hills beyond the city limits.

Francesco's final stop on his walking tour of Florence was the hilltop town of Fiesole, located just a few kilometers outside the city. As he hiked along the winding roads that lead up to the town, he encountered ancient Roman ruins, including a well-preserved amphitheater that dates back to the first century AD. When he reached the town's central piazza, he was greeted with stunning views of the Tuscan countryside and the surrounding hills, dotted with olive groves and vineyards. As he sat in a local cafe, sipping a cappuccino and nibbling on biscotti, Francesco felt a sense of tranquility and peace that he had never experienced before.

Upon returning to Florence, Francesco was determined to share his newfound discoveries with others. He started a walking tour company that focused on showing visitors the hidden treasures of the city, beyond the usual tourist hotspots. He also became an advocate for sustainable tourism, encouraging visitors to explore the city on foot or by bike, rather than relying on cars or buses that contribute to pollution and congestion.

Thanks to Francesco's efforts, Florence became known not just for its famous art and architecture but also for its hidden gems that only locals knew about. Visitors from around the world flocked to the city, eager to experience the magic of Florence through walking and discover the city's hidden treasures for

13. France: "A Journey of Self-Discovery Through Walking"

Sophie had always felt a bit disconnected from the natural world. She had grown up in Paris, surrounded by concrete and noise. But as she approached her thirties, she realized she needed a change. She wanted to reconnect with nature, explore her community, and discover recent places. So, she made a bold decision. She would leave her job, pack a small backpack, put on her hiking boots, and set off on a journey of self-discovery through walking.

Her first stop was the Loire Valley. She walked along the riverbanks, through the rolling hills, and past the vineyards. She stopped at small towns and villages, talked to the locals, and tasted the local food and wine. She felt free and alive, surrounded by nature and the beauty of the French countryside. But it wasn't always easy. Sometimes, she had to walk for hours under the scorching sun, with blisters on her feet and a heavy backpack on her shoulders. But the more she walked, the more she felt connected to the earth, to the sky, and to herself.

Next, she headed to the Pyrenees Mountains. She walked through the forests, up the hills, and across the streams. She camped in the wild and woke up to breathtaking views of the sunrise. She met other hikers and shared stories around the campfire. She felt connected to something bigger than herself, something spiritual and transformative. But it wasn't always safe. Once, she got lost in the fog, and it took her hours to find her way back to the trail. Another time, she had to run away from a pack of wild dogs. But the more she walked, the more she felt confident, resilient, and adventurous.

Finally, she arrived at the Mediterranean coast. She walked along the beaches, through the olive groves, and up the cliffs. She swam in the crystal-clear waters and watched the sunset over the sea. She felt grateful and humble, realizing how small she was in the grand scheme of things. But it was not always peaceful. Once, she got caught in a storm, and she had to find shelter in a cave. Another time, she got stung by a jellyfish, *and it took her a while to recover. But the more she walked, the more she felt grateful, curious, and open-minded.*

After three months of walking, Sophie returned to Paris. She was a changed person. She had found a new appreciation for nature, a deeper connection to her community, and a sense of adventure she never knew she had. She started a blog about her journey and inspired others to take their own walking adventures. She also volunteered for an environmental organization, helping to protect the natural beauty of the places she had visited. And she fell in love with a fellow hiker, who shared her passion for walking, nature, and life.

Positive Bonds: Health and Connection through Dog-Walking

14. Title: "Tales of Laughter and Leashes: The Adventures of Berlin's Dynamic Dog-Walking Duo"

Greta: "Lena, we seriously need to shake off this lethargy and embrace the wild world of exercise! I mean, we're practically moving in slow motion, like two sloths on a leisurely stroll through molasses."

Lena: laughing "You're right, Greta! It's like we've become the poster children for 'Couch Potatoes

Anonymous.' But how on earth do we morph into fitness enthusiasts overnight?"

Greta: "Fear not, Lena! I have concocted a master plan that involves harnessing the magical powers of our canine companions. We shall become... 'The Mighty Morning Dog-Walking Duo!'"

Lena: raising an eyebrow "Mighty, huh? Are we sure our dogs are on board with this? Max might just give us the side-eye and demand a raise in treats."

Greta: "Oh, they're on board, Lena! They've been secretly holding canine conferences, plotting how to get us off our butts. And trust me, they've even drafted a motivational speech for us in the language of enthusiastic tail wags."

Lena: giggling "Alright, then! I can see Luna rehearsing her motivational woofs in the mirror already."

Greta: "Excellent! And to ensure our success, we shall make an oath in the presence of these bewildered pigeons: 'We solemnly swear to chase away laziness, outwit the snooze button, and conquer the sidewalks like champions!'"

Lena: saluting dramatically "I pledge allegiance to the paws, and to the leashes, for which they stand, one team, under the morning sun, indivisible, with brisk walks and canine cuddles for all!"

Greta: bursting into laughter "That's the spirit, Lena! Now let's get ready to embrace the great outdoors like never before. And remember, if anyone asks why we're out here so early, we're conducting a top-secret mission to discover the hidden treasures of dewdrops."

Lena: "Ah, yes! The age-old quest for the mystical morning moisture! Our secret shall remain safe with the squirrels and the sparrows."

Greta: "And with that, Lena, we embark on an epic journey of epic proportions, destined to become the stuff of local legends. We'll go down in history as the pioneers of pet-powered perspiration!"

Lena: "I can already see the headlines: 'Dynamic Duo Discovers Uncharted Territories of Fresh Air and Unlocks Canine Enlightenment!'"

Greta: "And our dogs will be crowned as 'Knights of Wagging Tails,' bestowed with the highest honor: unlimited belly rubs."

Lena: "Greta, you've truly outdone yourself with this plan. Who knew that exercise could come with a side of side-splitting laughter?"

Greta: "Well, Lena, they say laughter is the best ab workout, so we're practically sculpting our six-packs with every giggle."

Lena: "And Luna and Max are the comedic coaches we never knew we needed!"

Greta: "Exactly! So, Lena, let the fitness frenzy and laughter extravaganza commence!"

And so, armed with their uproarious spirit and the unwavering support of their furry sidekicks, Greta and Lena embarked on a journey of fitness, friendship, and belly-aching laughter, turning each morning into an unforgettable comedic escapade in the heart of Berlin's Tiergarten Park. As they strolled beneath the lush canopies and amidst the whispers of the park's centuries-old trees, they couldn't help but recall the famous phrase, "All who wander are not lost," and indeed, they had found a path to joy and vitality that was as vibrant as the city around them.

15. Anna had been feeling unmotivated and aimless for months.

She was stuck in a rut, feeling like she was just going through the motions of her daily routine without any real purpose. She knew she needed to make a change, but she didn't know where to start.

One day, as she was walking home from work, she saw a woman walking her dog in the park. The woman looked so happy and content, and the dog was wagging its tail and bounding around in excitement. Anna felt a pang of envy - she had always loved animals, but she lived in a small apartment and didn't have the space or time to care for a pet.

But then she had an idea. What if she started walking dogs for other people? She could get some exercise, spend time with animals, and maybe even make some extra money. It seemed like the perfect solution to her problem.

She started looking for dog-walking jobs online, and soon enough she had a handful of clients. She would spend her mornings and afternoons walking dogs of all shapes and sizes, from tiny terriers to massive mastiffs. She found that the fresh air and exercise helped her feel more energized and focused, and she loved spending time with the dogs.

But the biggest change came when she realized that the dogs were holding her accountable. They depended on her to show up every day and take them for their walks. Even on days when she didn't feel like leaving the house, she knew she had to go out and walk the dogs. And once she was out there, she always felt better.

One of her regular clients was a golden retriever named Max. Max was a big, friendly dog who loved to play fetch and chase after squirrels. Whenever Anna walked Max, she felt like she was in a different world - a world where everything was simple and joyful. Max's tail would wag constantly, and he would nuzzle his nose into her hand whenever she stopped to pet him.

Walking with Max helped Anna to stay motivated and accountable in her own life. Whenever she felt lost or uncertain, she would think of Max and how happy he was just to be outside and exploring the world. And whenever she needed a little extra push to get out of bed in the morning, she would remember that Max was counting on her to show up and take him for a walk.

Over time, Anna found that her dog-walking business had become more than just a way to make some extra money. It had become a source of purpose and inspiration in her life. She felt like she was part of a community of animal lovers who were all striving to make the world a better place, one dog walk at a time. And she knew that as long as she had Max and the other dogs by her side, she could face whatever challenges came her way.

It's inspiring to see how Anna was able to find a sense of purpose and motivation through dog-walking. It's a great example of how small changes in our daily routine can have a big impact on our overall well-being.

Having a daily routine that includes physical activity, spending time in nature, and engaging with animals can be beneficial for both our physical and mental health. It can also provide a sense of structure and accountability that can help us stay motivated and focused on our goals.

In addition to the benefits of dog-walking, Anna's experience also highlights the importance of finding meaning and purpose in our lives. When we feel like we have a sense of purpose, we are more likely to feel motivated, engaged, and fulfilled.

Finding purpose can be a journey, and it may require some experimentation and exploration. But by being open to new experiences and following our passions, we can discover activities that bring us joy and a sense of meaning.

Overall, Anna's story is a reminder that sometimes the smallest changes can make the biggest difference in our lives. By taking a chance and trying something new, we may be able to unlock a source of motivation, purpose, and joy that we never knew was there.

Stroll Together, Thrive Together:
Walking with Loved Ones

16. Once upon a time, in the heart of Amsterdam, *there lived three friends - Mia, James, and Lisa. Mia was born in a charming old townhouse along one of the picturesque canals that crisscrossed the city. James hailed from a family with deep roots in Amsterdam, having been born in a cozy apartment overlooking a bustling square in the city center. Lisa's story began in a modern apartment building on the outskirts of Amsterdam, surrounded by green parks and serene lakes.*

They were all enthusiastic about living healthy and active lifestyles and would often go to the gym together. But recently, they had been struggling to stay motivated and accountable to their fitness goals.

Mia, being the proactive friend that she is, came up with an idea to help keep them on track. She suggested that they take a walk through the beautiful streets of Amsterdam, pointing out that it would be good for their mental health and would give them a chance to appreciate the stunning city that they lived in.

Initially, James and Lisa were hesitant, thinking that walking wouldn't be enough of a workout, but they eventually gave in and decided to try it. As they strolled through the city, they took in the beautiful canals, vibrant tulip fields, and stunning architecture. The sun was shining, and the cool breeze made it a perfect day for a walk.

As they walked, the three friends talked about their struggles with staying motivated and accountable to their fitness goals. They realized that they had been relying too much on each other to keep them on track and needed to find new ways to stay motivated.

That's when they came up with the idea of setting individual fitness goals and holding each other accountable. They decided to share their goals with each other and check in regularly to see how they were progressing. They also decided to try new activities together to keep things interesting and challenging.

Over the next few weeks, they stuck to their goals and supported each other every step of the way. They went on bike rides, tried yoga classes, and even went on a weekend hiking trip together. They found that by doing different activities and supporting each other, they were able to stay motivated and accountable to their fitness goals.

But it wasn't about fitness - the three friends found that their walks through Amsterdam had become a regular source of inspiration for them. They found joy in discovering new hidden spots, trying out new cafes and restaurants, and experiencing the unique culture of their city.

As they continued their walking tours of Amsterdam, they discovered that it wasn't about staying healthy, but it was also about nurturing their friendship and strengthening their bond. They realized that walking together had given them the opportunity to catch up and share stories, and that it was a special way to spend quality time together.

The more they walked, the more their bond grew, and the more motivated they became to stay active and healthy. They also started to invite other friends to join them on their walks, creating a wider community of like-minded people who were also looking to live their best lives.

In the end, their walking tours of Amsterdam had become a regular part of their lives. They had *discovered that it wasn't about the destination, but about the journey and the moments they shared together. They had found that even small steps can make a big difference and that having a supportive group of friends can make all the difference in achieving their goals.*

17. In the bustling heart of New York City, *a tale of transformation unfurled within the Johnson family, a family submerged in the frenzied currents of modern life. Amid the relentless symphony of honking horns and bustling sidewalks, the Johnsons found themselves ensnared in the clamor, their well-being an afterthought amidst the chaos.*

Yet, like alchemists of old, they sought to transmute the ordinary into the extraordinary, to infuse their lives with vitality that would radiate beyond their daily grind. A fervent desire was born—a desire to invigorate their existence, to breathe life into their mundane routine. Thus, their journey began a journey that would see them alight upon a path of renewal and shared enchantment.

In the glow of twilight, as the city's luminous tapestry began to unfold, the Johnsons gathered around their dining table, not just to nourish their bodies but to nourish their souls with candid conversation. A revelation dawned upon them—amid the whirlwind of obligations, their health had become a silent casualty. United by this realization, they yearned for metamorphosis.

Drawing from the essence of unity, the Johnsons chose a simple act that would symbolize their collective commitment—a family walk. The sidewalks of their neighborhood became their tapestry, and the streets, their canvas. The daily walk, a ritual, demanded courage; it was an invocation of shared dedication that transcended exhaustion. Each step became a brushstroke, painting a portrait of perseverance.

At the outset, the weight of the day clung to them, making each stride a testament to their resilience. But their pledge to one another fostered a force that propelled them forward. They traversed short distances at first, the concrete beneath their feet a conduit for stories and laughter. The city, once their backdrop, transformed into their playground.

As days flowed into weeks, their strides lengthened, mirroring the growth within. The symphony of their laughter intermingled with the city's melodies. No longer confined to their familiar streets, they ventured forth to explore the city's secrets—hidden parks, meandering trails—unveiling their home anew.

And so, as the sun dipped below the skyline each day, the Johnsons found solace in the rhythm of their footsteps. Vitality coursed through them, dispelling the weariness that once held sway. Their evenings became a tableau of shared stories and dreams, a sanctuary of laughter and mutual support. Their journey was not just physical; it was a voyage to the heart of kinship.

In unity, they found strength. The promise they made bound them to a shared purpose, an unwavering commitment to uplift each other. Adversities crumbled in the face of this bond—the rain's embrace, the siren call of procrastination—none could deter them. They held each other's aspirations close, intertwining their destinies in a pact unbreakable.

Within this odyssey, they discovered new milestones to conquer, new summits to ascend. Each step became a triumph, every obstacle a stepping stone. Fuelled by their newfound vitality, they embraced holistic wellness, nurturing their bodies with hydration and nourishment, mirroring the transformation within their souls.

Their daily walk metamorphosed into a sacred rite—a testament to their resilience, a tribute to their unity. Beyond physical health, it kindled a glow within them, an ember of harmony that warmed their relationships, strengthening their familial ties. Their *once-hectic lives now flowed to a different rhythm, a rhythm orchestrated by their unwavering commitment to each other and to themselves.*

In the grand tapestry of their existence, the Johnsons had woven a thread of determination, uniting their hearts and harmonizing their lives. They had embarked upon a journey fueled by accountability, breathing life into the mundane and rekindling the spark of imagination. And as they journeyed onward, they proved that through collective will, even the most profound alchemy is possible—a transformation that turns the ordinary into the extraordinary, a harmonious symphony composed by the echoes of their united steps.

Everyday Walkers: Conquering Obstacles, Achieving Success
Overcoming Obstacles: How Daily Walking Transformed Lives

18. Title: Walking Towards Success in Norway's Challenging Terrain

In the picturesque village of Nordlys nestled deep within the heart of Norway, a group of determined individuals discovered the transformative power of a simple yet powerful routine — walking. Despite the challenging weather and busy schedules, these individuals managed to turn walking into a daily ritual that not only improved their physical health but also brought them success in various aspects of life.

One such success story belonged to Elin Olsen, a middle-aged architect who had always struggled to find time for exercise amidst her demanding job and family responsibilities. Elin realized that she needed to make a change when her energy levels plummeted, and her creativity at work began to suffer. She decided to start walking every morning, even if it meant waking up an hour earlier. At first, the freezing temperatures and snow-covered paths were discouraging, but Elin's determination was unwavering. She invested in proper winter gear and found solace in the tranquil beauty of the snowy landscape. As weeks turned into months, Elin not only felt healthier but also found her mind brimming with innovative ideas for her architectural projects. Her colleagues and clients noticed the positive shift, and her career began to flourish.

Another inspiring tale emerged from the life of Lars Bergstrom, a retired fisherman who had always been active but had neglected regular exercise after retirement. Lars missed the camaraderie of the sea and the routine of his fishing days. One day, he decided to bring that routine back by walking along the village's rugged coastline. Rain or shine, Lars would be found walking with purpose, often collecting seashells and picking up litter along the way. His dedication caught the attention of the village's youth, who began to join him on his walks. Lars became a beloved figure, sharing tales of his fishing adventures while imparting wisdom about hard work and perseverance. The simple act of walking not only improved Lars' physical health but also gave him a renewed sense of purpose and connection with his community.

Nina Lindstrom, a young teacher, faced her own set of challenges. Her days were consumed by lesson planning and grading, leaving her with little time for herself. However, Nina recognized that self-care was crucial for her well-being and her ability to inspire her students. She started a walking club for her fellow teachers, organizing short walks during lunch breaks and longer hikes on weekends. The camaraderie of the group and the beauty of Norway's landscape made the walks a delightful escape from the daily grind. Nina's initiative spread throughout the school, leading to a positive shift in the overall work environment. Students also noticed their teachers' increased energy and enthusiasm, creating a ripple effect of inspiration within the school's walls.

In Nordlys, the success stories of Elin, Lars, and Nina became emblematic of the village's spirit – one that embraced challenges and turned them into *opportunities. Through their dedication to walking, they not only improved their physical health but also overcame obstacles, strengthened their communities, and achieved success in their respective endeavors. As word of their stories spread, more individuals in Norway were inspired to step out, regardless of the weather or time constraints, to experience the transformative power of a daily walk.*

19. Hiking Through the Shadows

Nestled deep within the heart of the majestic Appalachian Mountains, there exists a hidden gem known only as the "Path of Whispers." Its name, a whispered secret among nature enthusiasts, beckons to those souls yearning for adventure and self-discovery. Among the chosen few drawn by its enchanting allure is Mark, a man who has long battled the relentless specter of anxiety.

The mere thought of traversing the rugged terrain alone would have been unfathomable to Mark in the past. Yet, armed with nothing but his trusty backpack and a sturdy walking stick, he embarks on a transformative journey that will test the very limits of his spirit.

The trail reveals itself as a relentless rollercoaster of challenges – steep ascents that threaten to steal his breath away, treacherous descents that test the strength of his resolve, and the ever-present shroud of solitude that envelops him like a cloak. With each step, Mark's heart races, whether it's the thrill of encountering untamed wildlife or the awe-inspiring beauty that surrounds him.

Nights become a symphony of solitude, where the only lullabies are the whispers of the wind through the trees and the gentle rustle of leaves beneath his tent. Yet, amidst the darkness, there is a profound sense of peace—a quiet reassurance that he is exactly where he needs to be.

Emerging from weeks of solitude, Mark is a changed man. The once-imposing shadows of doubt that clouded his mind have now given way to the radiant light of accomplishment. His journey was not just about conquering the treacherous trail but, most importantly, about conquering the deep-seated fears that had held him captive for so long.

A Journey of Self-Discovery

Mark's triumphant return from the "Path of Whispers" marks the dawn of a new era in his life. While he has always been one to set ambitious goals for himself, this adventure has left an indelible mark on his soul. It's more than just conquering physical challenges; it's a testament to his unwavering determination to break through the mental barriers that have held him captive for years.

As he eases back into his everyday life, Mark can't help but reflect on the profound lessons he has gleaned from his time on the trail. It is here that he discovers the transformative power of pushing beyond his comfort zone. The solitude allows him to confront his anxieties head-on, and with every passing day, his confidence grows stronger.

Fueled by his own transformation, Mark feels a calling deep within his heart to share his story with others who are battling similar demons. He begins by becoming an active member of local hiking clubs and taking the lead on group excursions, offering his guidance and unwavering support to those in need. Nature, he believes, holds the key to healing, and he is determined to help others experience the same sense of triumph and renewal that has reshaped his own life.

Overcoming Obstacles

Mark's path to helping others is not without its hurdles. Skeptics doubt his ability to lead hiking groups, given his history of anxiety. Yet, Mark uses their doubts as fuel to stoke his determination. Each successful group hike becomes a testament to his resilience, inspiring others to break free from their own self-imposed limitations.

One of Mark's most challenging endeavors is assisting a young woman named Sarah. Sarah reaches out to him after hearing about his hiking group, confessing her crippling social anxiety and lifelong avoidance of the great outdoors. Mark sees in Sarah a reflection of his own past struggles, and he knows he has to help her overcome her fears, just as he has overcome his own.

With unwavering patience and compassion, Mark works alongside Sarah for months, starting with short walks in a nearby park and gradually progressing to more challenging trails. It's a slow and occasionally frustrating journey, but Mark's persistence never wanes. He shares his own stories of battling anxiety and reminds her that it's okay to take things one step at a time.

A Community of Triumph

With diligence and determination, Sarah eventually musters the courage to join one of Mark's group hikes. Her triumph isn't just a victory for her; it's a vindication of Mark's mission. Witnessing her radiant smile as she conquers her fears is a testament to the strength of human resolve and the profound impact of a supportive community.

Word of Mark's hiking group and its mission begins to spread. People from various walks of life, each *grappling with their unique challenges and anxieties, join the "Steps of Triumph" community. It blossoms into a diverse network of individuals all striving for personal triumphs, connected not only by their love for the outdoors but also by their shared journey towards self-discovery.*

As Mark continues to lead the group and share his story, he realizes that the "Path of Whispers" has led him not only to conquer his anxiety but also to discover the immense power of helping others find their own paths to triumph. Through the healing embrace of nature, unwavering determination, and the warmth of a supportive community, he has unearthed the true essence of achieving personal goals – it's about venturing beyond one's limits, both within and outside the self. It's about stepping into the light of a brighter, more triumphant future.

20. The Camino de Santiago, also known as the Way of Saint James, is an ancient pilgrimage route in northern Spain that leads to the city of Santiago de Compostela, where tradition holds that the remains of Saint James the Apostle are buried.

For more than a thousand years, pilgrims from all over the world have journeyed on foot or by bike to reach Santiago de Compostela. Marked by yellow arrows and shells, the route traverses rugged mountains, lush forests, and historic towns and villages. The Camino Francés, starting in Saint-Jean-Pied-de-Port, France, and spanning about 800 kilometers (500 miles) to Santiago de Compostela, is the most popular route. While completing the entire route typically takes four to six weeks, many opt to walk shorter sections or bike instead.

Beyond its spiritual significance, the Camino de Santiago is renowned for its natural beauty, cultural heritage, and sense of community. Pilgrims find rest, sustenance, and companionship in albergues, hostels along the way. The Camino has grown increasingly popular in recent years, attracting individuals seeking personal challenge, communion with nature, and cultural exploration.

As a child, I, Michael, harbored a deep desire to undertake the pilgrimage journey to Santiago de Compostela. The idea of walking the ancient route had always captivated me, and after years of dreaming, I finally resolved to embark on the adventure.

On a sunny spring morning, May 30, 1980, I departed from Zaragoza. My backpack held only the essentials: a change of clothes, toiletries, and a small notebook for jotting down thoughts and reflections.

The landscapes I encountered along the way were breathtaking. I passed through picturesque villages with old stone houses and churches, crossed rivers and streams, and climbed steep hills offering stunning views of the countryside.

It was during this journey that I encountered Sofia, prompting me to halt and offer my assistance. Patiently, I listened as she shared her fears and concerns, offering words of encouragement and support.

"Thank you," she said, smiling faintly. "I think I just need a break. I've been walking for hours, and I'm starting to feel a little overwhelmed."

I nodded in understanding. "I know the feeling," I replied. "This path may be tough, but it is also incredibly rewarding. Where are you from?"

"I'm from Brazil," Sofia said. "I decided to make this pilgrimage as a way to challenge myself and get in touch with my spirituality."

I was impressed. "That's amazing," I remarked. "I'm doing something similar, in a way. It's a powerful experience, isn't it?"

Sofia nodded, seeming grateful for the conversation. We walked together for a while, discussing our reasons for walking the Camino and sharing stories about our lives. I learned that Sofia was a nurse and had always been drawn to helping others, which explained her decision to undertake this challenging pilgrimage.

Approaching a steep hill, Sofia began to slow down. "I don't know if I'll make it up this hill," she confessed, panic evident in her voice.

Observing her struggle, I offered to carry her backpack. "It's the least I can do," I insisted. "We're all in this together, right?"

Sofia looked relieved and grateful. "Thank you," she said, her voice cracking with emotion. "I don't know what I would do without you."

As we ascended the hill together, I could see Sofia's determination despite her struggles. "You're doing great," I encouraged her. "Just take it one step at a time."

Finally reaching the summit, Sofia collapsed to the ground, breathing heavily. "Thank you," she said again, tears in her eyes. "I couldn't have done it without you."

Sitting beside her, I placed my hand on her shoulder. "We're all in this together," I reassured her. "We help each other; this is the Way."

Throughout our journey, Sofia and I developed a strong friendship. We walked side by side every day, sharing stories and supporting each other. As we approached the end of the pilgrimage, a sense of sadness enveloped me, knowing our time together was drawing to a close.

"I don't want this to end," Sofia confessed one day, while we sat in a cafe enjoying a coffee. "I feel like we've been through so much together."

It was on one of those sun-kissed afternoons, amid the rolling hills and quaint villages, that our journey took an unexpected turn. Approaching a rustic inn nestled along the trail, the lively chatter of fellow pilgrims beckoned us inside. Little did we know, destiny awaited in the form of Maurizio and Pipo.

Stepping into the inn, the aroma of hearty Spanish cuisine engulfed us, and the clinking of glasses filled the air. Our eyes met those of two friendly faces – Maurizio, with his infectious laughter and laid-back demeanor, and Pipo, whose Miami charm radiated with every word he spoke.

Seizing the moment, Sofia and I joined their table, initiating a conversation that would cement our friendship into the very fabric of our pilgrimage.

With a mischievous glint in his eyes, Maurizio remarked, "Hey there, fellow wanderers! What brings you to this corner of the world?"

Sofia and I exchanged glances, sharing a smile that revealed the purpose of our journey. "We're on the Camino de Santiago, seeking a deeper connection and a sense of purpose," I replied, the sincerity of our quest evident in my words.

Sipping on his glass of Rioja, Pipo chimed in, "Well, isn't that something? We're on the same path, my friends. Fate has a funny way of bringing kindred spirits together, doesn't it?"

And so, the evening unfolded in a symphony of laughter, shared stories, and newfound camaraderie. As we recounted tales of our lives and the paths that led us to the Camino, the inn's walls absorbed the essence of our connection.

Days turned into weeks, and our quartet navigated the challenges of the Camino together – the blisters, the exhaustion, and moments of pure, unfiltered joy. Maurizio's carefree spirit and Pipo's unwavering *optimism became integral parts of our pilgrimage, transforming mere acquaintances into lifelong friends.*

As we finally reached the majestic Cathedral of Santiago de Compostela, a profound sense of accomplishment washed over us. The journey had not only led us to the sacred destination but had also woven the threads of friendship tightly around our hearts.

Under the shadow of the cathedral, surrounded by the echoes of pilgrims past, our quartet stood united, forever connected by the serendipity of the Camino. As the sun dipped below the horizon, casting a golden glow over the historic city, we embraced the realization that our journey had not just been about reaching a destination but finding lifelong companions in Maurizio and Pipo – friends for the ages, forged on the trail of self-discovery and shared laughter.

CHAPTER 15:
"Globetrotter's Paradise: Unveiling Earth's Most Alluring Walking Trails"

There are countless beautiful places to walk around the world, but here are some of the most popular and breathtaking ones:

1. The Camino de Santiago, Spain - This ancient pilgrimage route through northern Spain offers stunning scenery, historic towns, and a unique cultural experience.

2. Cinque Terre, Italy - This rugged coastline is a UNESCO World Heritage site and offers stunning views of the Ligurian Sea, colorful villages, and scenic trails.

3. Banff National Park, Canada - With its crystal-clear lakes, snow-capped mountains, and lush forests, Banff offers some of the most beautiful hiking trails in the world.

4. Petra, Jordan - This ancient city carved into the rock offers incredible views and a unique glimpse into the history and culture of the Middle East.

5. Machu Picchu, Peru - The Incan ruins of Machu Picchu are nestled high in the Andes mountains, offering breathtaking views of the surrounding landscape.

6. The Great Ocean Walk, Australia - This coastal trail along the Great Ocean Road in Victoria offers stunning views of rugged cliffs, pristine beaches, and ocean vistas.

7. Yosemite National Park, USA - With its towering granite cliffs, giant sequoias, and cascading waterfalls, Yosemite is one of the most beautiful and awe-inspiring natural landscapes in the world.

8. The Scottish Highlands, Scotland - With their dramatic mountains, tranquil lochs, and wild landscapes, the Scottish Highlands offer some of the most scenic walking routes in Europe.

9. The Inca Trail, Peru - This ancient trail winds through the Andes Mountains to the famous ruins of Machu Picchu, offering breathtaking views and a unique cultural experience.

10. The Milford Track, New Zealand - Known as the "finest walk in the world," the Milford Track takes hikers through stunning fiords, mountains, and valleys in the remote wilderness of New Zealand's South Island.

1. The Camino de Santiago, also known as the Way of Saint James, is an ancient pilgrimage route in northern Spain that leads to the city of Santiago de Compostela, where the remains of Saint James the Apostle are said to be buried.

2. Cinque Terre is a beautiful and unique stretch of coastline located in the Liguria region of Italy. It is made up of five small towns - Monterosso al Mare, Vernazza, Corniglia, Manarola, and Riomaggiore - that are nestled along the rugged Mediterranean coast.

The Cinque Terre region is known for its colorful buildings, winding streets, and dramatic scenery. The towns are connected by a network of hiking trails that offer breathtaking views of the Ligurian Sea and the surrounding hillsides. These trails are part of the Cinque Terre National Park, which is a UNESCO World Heritage Site and a protected area that aims to preserve the natural and cultural heritage of the region.

The hiking trails in Cinque Terre range in difficulty, from easy walks through vineyards and olive groves to more challenging climbs up steep hillsides. Some of the most popular trails include the Blue Trail, which connects all five towns and offers stunning views of the coastline, and the Sentiero Azzurro, which is a shorter trail that connects Riomaggiore and Manarola.

In addition to hiking, Cinque Terre is also known for its delicious seafood, wine, and local specialties such as pesto and focaccia. The towns are filled with restaurants, cafes, and bars that offer a range of traditional Italian dishes and local delicacies.

3. Banff National Park, Canada - With its crystal-clear lakes, snow-capped mountains, and lush forests, Banff offers some of the most beautiful hiking trails in the world.

Banff National Park is a vast wilderness area located in the Canadian Rockies, in the province of Alberta, Canada. It is one of the most beautiful national parks in the world, known for its pristine landscapes, crystal-clear lakes, and snow-capped mountains.

The park covers an area of over 6,600 square kilometers (2,500 square miles) and offers a range of hiking trails that cater to all skill levels, from easy walks to challenging backcountry treks. The trails are well-marked and offer stunning views of the surrounding landscapes, including glaciers, waterfalls, and forests.

Some of the most popular hikes in Banff National Park include the Plain of Six Glaciers Trail, which offers incredible views of glaciers, and the Lake Agnes Tea House Trail, which leads to a historic tea house overlooking a beautiful mountain lake. The park also offers several multi-day backpacking trips, such as the Skyline Trail, which takes hikers on a high-elevation journey through the park's rugged backcountry.

In addition to hiking, Banff National Park is also known for its wildlife, including bears, elk, moose, and wolves. Visitors can also enjoy a range of outdoor activities such as skiing, snowshoeing, canoeing, and kayaking.

The park has several developed areas for visitors, including the town of Banff, which offers a range of accommodation options, restaurants, and shops. The park is also home to several natural hot springs, which provide a relaxing way to unwind after a day of hiking or other activities.

4. Petra, Jordan - This ancient city carved into the rock offers incredible views and a unique glimpse into the history and culture of the Middle East.

Petra is an ancient city located in the southwestern region of Jordan, known for its unique architecture and breathtaking natural surroundings. The city was carved into the rock by the Nabataeans, an ancient Arab tribe, over 2,000 years ago and was an important center of trade and culture.

The most famous structure in Petra is the Treasury, which is carved out of a sandstone cliff and features intricate carvings and ornate details. The city is also home to a range of other impressive structures, such as the Royal Tombs, the Monastery, and the Roman Theater, which provide a glimpse into the city's rich history and cultural heritage.

In addition to its architectural wonders, Petra is surrounded by stunning natural landscapes, including rugged mountains, deep gorges, and expansive deserts. Visitors can hike through the city and explore its many hidden corners or take a camel or horseback ride to explore the surrounding desert.

Petra is also known for its vibrant culture, with a rich mix of Arab, Bedouin, and other cultural influences. Visitors can enjoy traditional Bedouin music and dance performances, sample local cuisine, and learn about the history and traditions of the region.

5. Picchu is nestled high in the Andes mountains, offering breathtaking views of the surrounding landscape.

Machu Picchu is an ancient Incan city located high in the Andes Mountains of Peru, near the city of Cusco. The site was built in the 15th century, during the height of the Incan Empire, and was abandoned just over 100 years later, following the arrival of the Spanish conquistadors.

Today, Machu Picchu is one of the most popular tourist destinations in South America, attracting hundreds of thousands of visitors each year. The site is renowned for its stunning setting, perched on a high ridge overlooking the Urubamba River and surrounded by towering peaks and deep valleys.

The ruins of Machu Picchu include a range of impressive structures, including temples, terraced fields, and palaces, all built with intricate stonework and engineering. Visitors can hike through the site and explore its many hidden corners or take a guided tour to learn more about the history and significance of the ruins.

In addition to the ruins themselves, Machu Picchu is surrounded by stunning natural landscapes, including rugged mountains, deep valleys, and lush forests. Visitors can hike along the famous Inca Trail, which winds its way through the mountains and offers breathtaking views of the surrounding scenery.

6. The Great Ocean Walk, Australia - This coastal trail along the Great Ocean Road in Victoria offers stunning views of rugged cliffs, pristine beaches, and ocean vistas.

The Great Ocean Walk is a spectacular coastal trail located along the Great Ocean Road in Victoria, Australia. The trail covers a distance of approximately 100 kilometers and winds its way through rugged cliffs, pristine beaches, and stunning ocean vistas.

The Great Ocean Walk offers hikers the opportunity to experience some of the most breathtaking coastal scenery in Australia. Along the trail, visitors can take in the stunning views of the Southern Ocean and explore a range of unique geological formations, including the

Twelve Apostles, a series of limestone rock formations rising from the ocean.

The trail is divided into sections, allowing hikers to customize their journey and choose the length and difficulty of their hike. Along the way, visitors can enjoy a range of experiences, including wildlife spotting, beachcombing, and exploring charming coastal towns.

The Great Ocean Walk is also home to a range of flora and fauna, including rare and endangered species such as the southern right whale and the orange-bellied parrot. Hikers can experience the unique natural beauty of the region while also learning about the local ecology and conservation efforts.

7. Yosemite National Park, USA - With its towering granite cliffs, giant sequoias, and cascading waterfalls, Yosemite is one of the most beautiful and awe-inspiring natural landscapes in the world.

Yosemite National Park is a vast wilderness area located in the Sierra Nevada Mountains of California, USA. It is renowned for its awe-inspiring natural beauty, which includes towering granite cliffs, ancient giant sequoia trees, and cascading waterfalls.

The park covers an area of over 1,100 square miles and offers a range of outdoor recreational activities, including hiking, camping, rock climbing, and wildlife watching. Some of the most popular attractions in Yosemite include Half Dome, El Capitan, Yosemite Falls, and the Mariposa Grove of giant sequoias.

One of the most famous hikes in Yosemite is the Mist Trail, which takes visitors past Vernal and Nevada Falls, providing stunning views of the surrounding landscape. Another popular hike is the Half Dome Trail, which takes hikers to the summit of Half Dome, a towering granite peak that offers breathtaking views of the park.

In addition to its natural beauty, Yosemite is also home to a rich cultural history, with a long tradition of Native American habitation and a history of exploration and settlement. Visitors can learn about the park's cultural heritage at the Yosemite Museum and the Indian Village of Ahwahnee.

8. The Scottish Highlands, Scotland - With their dramatic mountains, tranquil lochs, and wild landscapes, the Scottish Highlands offer some of the most scenic walking routes in Europe. Absolutely! The Scottish Highlands are a rugged and beautiful region of Scotland that offer a wide variety of stunning walking routes. The area is known for its dramatic mountains, tranquil lochs, and wild landscapes, making it a popular destination for hikers and outdoor enthusiasts.

One of the most popular hiking routes in the Scottish Highlands is the West Highland Way, which covers approximately 154 kilometers and takes hikers through some of the most stunning landscapes in Scotland. The route passes through rolling hills, tranquil lochs, and rugged mountains, including Ben Nevis, the highest mountain in the British Isles.

Another popular hiking route in the Scottish Highlands is the Great Glen Way, which follows the Caledonian Canal and takes hikers from Fort William to Inverness. Along the way, visitors can take in stunning views of Loch Ness and the surrounding mountains, as well as experience the local wildlife and culture.

The Scottish Highlands are also home to a range of unique and beautiful natural landmarks, including the Isle of Skye, the Glenfinnan Viaduct, and the Falls of Foyers. Visitors can also explore charming villages and towns, sample local cuisine and whiskey, and learn about the region's rich cultural history.

9. The Inca Trail, Peru - This ancient trail winds through the Andes Mountains to the famous ruins of Machu Picchu, offering breathtaking views and a unique cultural experience.
Certainly! Mountains in Peru, leading hikers to the ancient Incan ruins of Machu Picchu. This route is

known for its stunning mountain scenery and rich cultural history, making it one of the most popular hiking destinations in the world.

The Inca Trail is an approximately 42-kilometer route that typically takes hikers four days to complete. Along the way, hikers will pass through a variety of different landscapes, including high-altitude mountain passes, lush rainforests, and ancient Incan ruins.

One of the most famous sites along the Inca Trail is the ruins of Wiñay Wayna, a spectacular Incan site that features terraces, fountains, and stone staircases. Other notable sites along the trail include the ruins of Runkurakay, Sayacmarca, and Phuyupatamarca.

The final destination of the Inca Trail is the world-famous ruins of Machu Picchu, a UNESCO World Heritage site that was built in the 15th century and is considered one of the most impressive archaeological sites in the world. The ruins are situated on a high mountain ridge overlooking the Sacred Valley and offer breathtaking views of the surrounding landscape.

10. The Milford Track, New Zealand - Known as the "finest walk in the world," the Milford Track takes hikers through stunning fiords, mountains, and valleys in the remote wilderness of New Zealand's South Island.

Absolutely! The Milford Track is one of the most popular and well-known hiking routes in the world and is considered by many to be the "finest walk in the world." The trail takes hikers through some of the most stunning natural landscapes in New Zealand's South Island, including rugged mountains, deep valleys, and stunning fiords.

The Milford Track is a 53.5-kilometer route that typically takes hikers four days to complete. The trail begins at Glade Wharf on the shores of Lake Te Anau and winds its way through some of the most breathtaking scenery in the region. Along the way, hikers will encounter a variety of different landscapes, including rainforests, alpine meadows, and glacier-carved valleys.

One of the highlights of the Milford Track is the stunning Mackinnon Pass, which rises to an elevation of 1,154 meters and offers breathtaking views of the surrounding landscape. The pass is named after Quintin Mackinnon, a legendary guide who first explored the area in the late 19th century.

Other notable sites along the Milford Track include the Clinton River, which flows through a deep, glacier-carved valley, and the stunning Sutherland Falls, which cascade down from an elevation of 580 meters and are considered one of the tallest waterfalls in the world.

CHAPTER 16:
Appendix

1. Famous walkers Throughout History
2. Sample Walking Plans
3. Glossary of Walking Terms

1. Famous walkers Throughout History

While the concept of "famous walkers" may not be as widely recognized as other historical figures, there are individuals known for their remarkable journeys on foot or their contributions to walking culture. Here are a few notable walkers throughout history:

John Muir (1838–1914):

Known as the "Father of the National Parks," Muir was a naturalist and environmentalist who walked extensively through the wilderness, advocating for the preservation of natural landscapes. His love for walking and nature inspired many.

Peace Pilgrim (1908–1981):

Peace Pilgrim, born Mildred Lisette Norman, was a woman who walked across the United States for nearly 30 years, spreading a message of peace. She walked more than 25,000 miles with no money and no possessions, relying on the kindness of strangers.

Patrick Leigh Fermor (1915–2011):

A British author and travel writer, Fermor is renowned for his long walk from the Netherlands to

Constantinople (Istanbul) in the 1930s. His journey was later documented in the books "A Time of Gifts" and "Between the Woods and the Water."

Christopher Hitchens (1949–2011):

The late British-American author and journalist was known for his intellectual pursuits. Hitchens undertook a famous walk from London to Oxford in 2000, documented in his book **"The Portable Atheist."**

Robyn Davidson (born 1950):

An Australian writer known for her memoir "Tracks," which details her solo 1,700-mile trek across the Australian desert with her dog and four camels. The journey was later adapted into a film.

Bill Bryson (born 1951):

While Bryson is primarily a humorist and travel writer, his book "A Walk in the Woods" recounts his attempt to hike the Appalachian Trail, providing a humorous and insightful perspective on long-distance hiking.

Nellie Bly (1864–1922):

Nellie Bly was an American journalist who, in 1889, attempted to replicate the fictional journey described in Jules Verne's "Around the World in Eighty Days." Bly completed her trip in just 72 days, making her a pioneer in circumnavigation.

Edward Payson Weston (1839–1929):
Weston, an American pedestrian, was a professional long-distance walker known for his feats in the late 19th and early 20th centuries. He gained fame for his transcontinental walks, including one from New York to San Francisco.

Plato (c. 428–348 BCE):
The ancient Greek philosopher Plato was known for his habit of engaging in long, contemplative walks. It's said that he founded the Academy, one of the earliest institutions of higher learning, where philosophical discussions often took place during walks in the groves.

Paul Salopek (born 1962):
An American journalist and author, Salopek is known for his ambitious project called the "Out of Eden Walk." He has been walking across the world, tracing the migration route of early humans, and documenting his journey for National Geographic.

Cheryl Strayed (born 1968):
The author of "Wild: From Lost to Found on the Pacific Crest Trail," Cheryl Strayed embarked on a solo journey of self-discovery by hiking over 1,000 miles on the Pacific Crest Trail. Her memoir recounts the challenges and personal growth experienced during her hike.

Jean-Jacques Rousseau (1712–1778):

The French philosopher Rousseau was known for his love of nature and walking. His book "Confessions" includes reflections on the importance of solitary walks for contemplation and inspiration.

Alfred Wainwright (1907–1991):

Wainwright was an English fellwalker, guidebook author, and illustrator. He is best known for his series of pictorial guides to the Lakeland fells, which have inspired countless walkers to explore the Lake District in England.

Hector Del Chiaro Capella (1911-1973):

author, explorer, journalist, and writer born in Barranquilla, Colombia, of Italian origins, is known for his adventure of walking from Barranquilla to New York. This journey lasted for two years, during which he was accompanied by three friends and three donkeys. He chronicled this experience in the book "Two Years Across America."

Amanda Walkins (born 1981):

An author and blogger, Amanda Walkins is known for her adventure of walking around the entire island of Anguilla in the Caribbean. Her journey, documented in the book "Caribbean Freedom," explores the beauty and challenges of the island.

Alexandra David-Néel (1868–1969):
A French-Belgian explorer, writer, and Buddhist, David-Néel was the first European woman to enter the forbidden city of Lhasa in Tibet. Her extensive travels, including long periods of walking in the Himalayas, are chronicled in her book "My Journey to Lhasa."

These individuals have left their mark on history through their remarkable walks, whether for exploration, personal growth, or philosophical contemplation.

2. Sample Walking Plans

Here are a few sample walking plans that cater to different fitness levels and goals. Before starting any new exercise routine, it's advisable to consult with a healthcare professional or personal trainer, especially if you have any existing health conditions.

Beginner Walking Plan:
Weeks 1-2: Getting Started
Monday-Friday: 10 minutes of brisk walking
Saturday: Rest or light activity (e.g., gentle stretching)
Sunday: 15 minutes of easy-paced walking
Weeks 3-4: Building Endurance

Monday-Friday: 15 minutes of brisk walking
Saturday: Rest or light activity
Sunday: 20 minutes of easy-paced walking

Weeks 5-6: Increasing Duration

Monday-Friday: 20 minutes of brisk walking
Saturday: Rest or light activity
Sunday: 25 minutes of easy-paced walking

Intermediate Walking Plan:
Weeks 1-2: Moderate Intensity
Monday-Friday: 30 minutes of brisk walking
Saturday: Rest or light activity
Sunday: 40 minutes of easy-paced walking
Weeks 3-4: Introducing Intervals

Monday: 30 minutes (alternating between 3 minutes brisk, 2 minutes easy)
Tuesday: 35 minutes of steady-paced walking
Wednesday: Rest or light activity
Thursday: 30 minutes (alternating between 3 minutes brisk, 2 minutes easy)
Friday: 40 minutes of easy-paced walking
Saturday: Rest or light activity
Sunday: 45 minutes of steady-paced walking
Weeks 5-6: Building Speed and Distance

Monday: 35 minutes (alternating between 4 minutes brisk, 2 minutes easy)
Tuesday: 40 minutes of steady-paced walking
Wednesday: Rest or light activity

Thursday: 35 minutes (alternating between 4 minutes brisk, 2 minutes easy)
Friday: 50 minutes of easy-paced walking
Saturday: Rest or light activity
Sunday: 60 minutes of steady-paced walking

Advanced Walking Plan:
Weeks 1-2: High-Intensity Intervals
Monday: 40 minutes (alternating between 5 minutes brisk, 2 minutes fast-paced)
Tuesday: 45 minutes of steady-paced walking
Wednesday: Rest or light activity
Thursday: 40 minutes (alternating between 5 minutes brisk, 2 minutes fast-paced)
Friday: 60 minutes of easy-paced walking
Saturday: Rest or light activity
Sunday: 75 minutes of steady-paced walking
Weeks 3-4: Increased Intensity and Distance

Monday: 50 minutes (alternating between 6 minutes brisk, 3 minutes fast-paced)
Tuesday: 60 minutes of steady-paced walking
Wednesday: Rest or light activity
Thursday: 50 minutes (alternating between 6 minutes brisk, 3 minutes fast-paced)
Friday: 75 minutes of easy-paced walking
Saturday: Rest or light activity
Sunday: 90 minutes of steady-paced walking

Remember to listen to your body, stay hydrated, and adjust the intensity as needed. Progression can be gradual, and it's essential to enjoy the process. If you experience pain or discomfort, **it's advisable to consult with a fitness professional or healthcare provider.**

3. Glossary of Walking Terms
1. **Active Commuting:**
   - Walking as a means of transportation to work or other destinations.
2. **Barefoot Walking:**
   - Walking without shoes, either on natural surfaces or specially designed areas.
3. **Blister Prevention:**
   - Techniques and products used to avoid the formation of blisters during walking.
4. **Brisk Walking:**
   - Walking at a faster pace than a leisurely stroll, often used for cardiovascular exercise.
5. **Cadence:**
   - The number of steps per minute taken during walking.

6. **Callus:**
   - Thickened and toughened skin on the feet, often caused by repeated friction during walking.
7. **Cane Fu:**
   - A form of exercise that combines walking with self-defense techniques using a cane.
8. **Cool Down:**
   - A period of light exercise and stretching after a walk to gradually lower the heart rate and prevent stiffness.
9. **CoolMax:**
   - A type of moisture-wicking fabric used in walking and athletic clothing to keep the body dry.
10. **Cooling Towel:**
    - A specialized towel designed to stay cool when wet, used to cool down during or after a walk.
11. **Dog Walking:**
    - Walking with a pet dog, often for exercise and companionship.
12. **Ergonomics:**
    - The study of how the design of tools and equipment affects human efficiency and well-being.

13. **Foot Arch:**
  - The curved area along the bottom of the foot that helps distribute body weight during walking.

14. **Footstrike:**
  - The manner in which the foot makes contact with the ground during each step.

15. **Gait:**
  - The manner or style of walking, including the movement of the arms and legs.

16. **Gait Analysis:**
  - The examination of an individual's walking pattern to assess biomechanics and identify issues.

17. **Gorp (Good Old Raisins and Peanuts):**
  - A high-energy trail mixes often consumed during long walks or hikes.

18. **HIIT Walking (High-Intensity Interval Training):**
  - Incorporating short bursts of intense walking with periods of lower-intensity walking or rest.

19. **Hiking:**
  - Walking outdoors, usually on trails, for recreational purposes and often involving more challenging terrain.

20. **Inclinometer:**
   - A device used to measure the incline or slope of a walking surface.

21. **Interval Walking:**
   - Alternating between periods of faster-paced walking and slower-paced walking or rest.

22. **MapMyWalk by Under Armour:**
   - An app for tracking walks, providing route planning, and offering a community of walkers.

23. **Metatarsalgia:**
   - Pain and inflammation in the ball of the foot, often associated with walking.

24. **Mobility Aids:**
   - Devices like canes or walking sticks used for support and stability during walking.

25. **Nordic Walking:**
   - A full-body exercise that involves walking with specialized poles, promoting upper body engagement.

26. **Orthotics:**
   - Customized shoe inserts designed to provide additional support and correct specific foot issues.

27. **Outdoor Fitness Trail:**
- A trail equipped with exercise stations for a combination of walking and fitness activities.

28. **Overpronation:**
- Excessive inward rolling of the foot during walking, which can affect gait and cause strain.

29. **Pace:**
- The speed at which a person walks, often measured in minutes per mile or kilometers per hour.

30. **Pedometer:**
- A device used to count the number of steps taken, often worn on the waist or carried in a pocket.

31. **Perambulator (Pram) Walking:**
- Walking while pushing a baby stroller or pram.

32. **Plogging:**
- A combination of jogging and picking up litter during walks or runs.

33. **Power Walking:**
- A faster-paced form of walking, involving exaggerated arm movements and purposeful strides.

34. **Reflective Gear:**
   - Clothing or accessories with reflective materials for visibility during low-light conditions.
35. **Rain Gear:**
   - Waterproof or water-resistant clothing and accessories for walking in the rain.
36. **Shoe Inserts (Insoles):**
   - Cushioned inserts placed inside shoes for added comfort and support during walking.
37. **Shoe Rotation:**
   - Alternating between different pairs of walking shoes to prevent wear and tear.
38. **Strava:**
   - A social fitness app that allows users to track and share their walking activities.
39. **Stride Frequency:**
   - The number of steps taken in a given time, often measured in steps per minute.
40. **Stride Length:**
   - The distance covered in a single step or stride while walking.
41. **Strava:**
   - A social fitness app that allows users to track and share their walking activities.

42. **Terrain:**

- The type of ground or landscape walked on, such as flat, hilly, or rocky terrain.

43. **Thermoregulation:**

- The body's ability to regulate its temperature, important during walks in varying weather conditions.

44. **Trail Walking:**

- Walking on natural paths or trails, often in parks or wooded areas.

45. **Treadmill Walking:**

- Walking on a stationary treadmill machine for exercise.

46. **Virtual Walking Challenge:**

- A challenge where participants virtually log walking miles to reach a specific destination or achieve a goal.

47. **Walkability:**

- The measure of how friendly an area is to walking, often considering factors like sidewalks, pedestrian paths, and safety.

48. **Walkable Community Design:**

- Urban planning that prioritizes pedestrian-friendly environments, encouraging walking.

49. Walk and Talk Therapy:

- A therapeutic approach where individuals engage in counseling sessions while walking.

50. Walking and Talk Therapy:

- A therapeutic approach where individuals engage in counseling sessions while walking.

51. Walking Accessibility:

- The ease with which people, including those with disabilities, can walk in a particular area.

52. Walking Challenge App:

- Mobile applications that encourage users to set and achieve walking goals.

53. Walking Club:

- A group of individuals who gather regularly to walk together for fitness and socialization.

54. Walking Desk:

- A desk designed to be used while walking on a treadmill, promoting movement during work.

55. Walking Economy:

- The energy efficiency of an individual's walking pattern.

56. **Walking Event:**

- Organized events, such as charity walks or marathons, where participants walk together for a cause.

57. **Walking Festival:**

- An organized event celebrating walking, often featuring guided walks and activities.

58. **Walking History Tour:**

- A guided walk that explores historical sites and provides insights into local history.

59. **Walking Interval Timer:**

- A tool or app that helps individuals time intervals for different walking intensities.

60. **Walking Marathon:**

- An organized event where participants walk a marathon distance (26.2 miles or 42.195 kilometers).

61. **Walking Meditation:**

- A mindfulness practice that involves walking slowly and deliberately, often in a meditative environment.

62. **Walking Meditation Group:**

- A group that practices walking meditation together, often led by a guide.

63. Walking Meditation Retreat:

- An organized event where participants engage in extended periods of walking meditation.

64. Walking Path:

- A designated route or trail for walking, often found in parks or recreational areas.

65. Walking Playlist:

- A curated list of music or audio content to accompany and motivate during walks.

66. Walking School Bus:

- A group of children walking to school with adult supervision in a structured manner.

67. Walking Score:

- A measure that assesses the walkability of a neighborhood or location based on proximity to amenities.

68. Walking Scorecard:

- A personal or community-based assessment of walking habits and achievements.

69. Walking Shoes:

- Footwear designed specifically for walking, providing comfort, support, and cushioning.

70.

71. **Walking Stick Insect:**
- An insect that mimics the appearance of a twig or walking stick for camouflage.

72. **Walking Stick (Trekking Pole):**
- A pole used for stability and support during walking, particularly in challenging terrains.

73. **Walk Score:**
- A measure that assesses the walkability of a neighborhood or location based on proximity to amenities.

74. **Walking Journal:**
- A diary or log where individuals can record their walking progress, routes, and experiences.

75. **Walking the Labyrinth:** A meditative practice involving walking a winding path leading to a center point.

76. **Urban Walking:**
- Walking within city or town environments, often for commuting or exploring urban landscapes.

Dear Reader,

As you conclude "The Longevity Benefits of Walking," we extend our heartfelt thanks for accompanying us on this enlightening journey. Walking is not just a physical activity; it is a path to enhanced well-being, vitality, and longevity.

Through the pages of this book, we have explored the myriad ways in which walking can positively impact your health and quality of life. From strengthening your cardiovascular system to boosting mental clarity and emotional balance, every step you take contributes to a healthier, happier you.

We hope that the insights, tips, and strategies shared here have inspired you to integrate walking into your daily routine and experience its transformative benefits firsthand. Whether you're strolling through nature's beauty or navigating city streets, every walk you take is a step towards a brighter, more vibrant future.

We would like to express our gratitude to all the readers who have devoted their time and attention to this book. Your curiosity, dedication to self-improvement, and commitment to holistic well-being are truly commendable. Remember that your journey towards better health and longevity is ongoing, and each step forward is a victory worth celebrating.

May your path be filled with health, happiness, and the simple joy of walking.

With gratitude,

Michael Luxiey

AUTHOR BIO

Michael Luxiey is an esteemed author, seasoned traveler, dedicated blogger, and a recognized expert in the field of longevity. With over five decades of exploring the globe, he has ventured through numerous countries, seeking and studying the most effective methods to lead a prolonged and fulfilling life. Currently residing in Ikaria, Greece, and Sardinia, Michael has immersed himself in the cultures renowned for their longevity and wellness practices.

Drawing from his extensive experiences and research, Michael has authored a series of insightful books focusing on longevity, optimal living, and nutrition. His notable works include **"The Longevity Bible,"** a comprehensive guide to extending and enhancing life quality, and **"The Longevity Kitchen,"** which delves into the relationship between diet and longevity.

His latest publication, **"The Longevity Benefits of Walking,"** presents a compelling exploration of the profound impact that walking can have on health, longevity, and overall well-being. Through this book, Michael Luxiey shares invaluable insights and practical strategies for integrating the benefits of walking into daily life, empowering readers to embark on a journey towards a healthier and more vibrant existence.

With his wealth of knowledge and passion for promoting wellness, Michael Luxiey continues to inspire individuals worldwide to embrace a lifestyle that fosters longevity, vitality, and joy.